Dragonflies and Pest Management

THE AUTHORS

Dr. Sathe Tukaram Vithalrao [M.Sc., Ph.D., Sangit Visharad, IBT (Seri.), F.S.E.Sc., F.I.S.E.C.], Professor in Entomology, Department of Zoology, Shivaji University, Kolhapur has teaching experience of 22 years in entomology. He is contributory teacher for M.Sc. courses in Department of Agrochemicals, Pest Management and Sericulture. He has published 165 research papers and 22 books *viz., Preet Patangachi* (drama, 1981), *Crop Protection from Insects* (Marathi), *Sericultural Crop Protection* (1998), *Biological Pest Control* (2000), *Cotton Pests and Biocontrol Agents* (2001), *Insect Pest Predators* (2001), *Sericulture and Pest Management* (2001), *Agrochemicals and Pest Management* (2003), *Insect Predators and Pest Management* (2003), *Vermiculture and Organic Farming* (2004), *Basic Entomology* (2005), *Fundamentals of Beekeeping* (2006), *Forest Entomology: A Textbook* (2008), etc. He guided 15 Ph.D. students, completed 4 major research projects (from CSIR, UST, UGC). He visited Canada (1988), Japan (1988), Thailand (2002, 2004), Spain (2005), France (2005), South Korea (2006), Nepal (2007) for academic work. He is member of editorial board of several journals in India and involved in T.V. programming of butterflies and moths. He has published several popular articles in daily newspapers and delivered talks through All India Radio. He got several prestigious awards "Environmentalists of the Year-2003", "Bharat Jyoti Award-2006", "Jewel of India Award-2006", Lifetime Education Achievement Award-2006", "Lifetime Achievement Award-2007", "International Gold Star Award-2007", "Eminent Citizen of India Award-2007" etc. He also got fellowships from several scientific societies.

Dr. K.P. Shinde (M.Sc., Ph.D.) is Lecturer in DKASC College, Ichalkaranji, Dist. Kolhapur. He has published twelve research papers in reputed journals. He has presented several research papers in national and international conferences/workshops/etc. He visited Spain and France in 2005 for academic work. He is life member of NESA, New Delhi and associated with local NGOs.

Dragonflies and Pest Management

Dr. T.V. Sathe
Entomology Division
Department of Zoology,
Shivaji University, Kolhapur, M.S.
(E-mail: drtvsathe@rediffmail.com
&
Dr. K.P. Shinde
Department of Zoology,
DKASC College, Ichalkaranji, M.S.

2016
Daya Publishing House®
A Division of
Astral International Pvt. Ltd.
New Delhi - 110 002

ISBN: 978-93-5124-003-7 (International Edition)

Published by : **Daya Publishing House®**
A Division of
Astral International Pvt. Ltd.
– ISO 9001:2008 Certified Company –
4760-61/23, Ansari Road, Darya Ganj
New Delhi-110 002
Ph. 011-43549197, 23278134
E-mail: info@astralint.com
Website: www.astralint.com

Preface

Dragonflies belong to Order-Odonata containing 600 species all over the world and considered as one of the largest and oldest winged insects, appeared about 350 million years ago. They are widely distributed throughout the world except in the extremely cold regions like Antarctica and Northern pole. The dragonflies are beautiful coloured insects and associated with water bodies such as ponds, lakes, dams, rivers, rice fields and all other types of wetlands. The dragonflies are very potential biocontrol agents of insect importance in integrated pest management, as biological pest control is pollution free and ecofriendly.

The book contains four chapters. First chapter deals with biodiversity of dragonflies to be utilized in biological pest control. In all 15 new species of dragonflies have been described and 6 species redescribed. Second chapter refers to biology of dragonflies which highlights life cycle, fecundity, habitat, behaviour, migration and endangered species. This information is extremely useful for mass rearing of dragonflies to be utilized in biological pest control. The chapter third is devoted for utilization of dragonflies in biological control of insect pests. It contains predator prey index of dragonflies, mass rearing techniques of dragonflies, methods of biological pest control and bicontrol programmes designed with dragonflies. This information will be helpful for undertaking biocontrol programmes of mosquito species and paddy pests in addition to other pests. The present work will fulfil the gap of information on dragonflies to be utilized in biological pest control programmes and will be stimulatory and helpful guide to students, teachers, farmers, scientists and industrialists working in the field of biological pest control.

T.V. Sathe

K.P. Shinde

Contents

Chapter 1

Biodiversity of Dragonflies

Diversity is the variability among living organisms from all sources, including terrestrial, marine and other aquatic ecosystems and the ecological complexes of which they are a part; this includes diversity within species, between species and of eco-system. Biodiversity is the species richness of plants, animals and micro-organisms, including their genetic make-up and the communities they form. Biodiversity has three components, *viz.* genetic, organismal and ecological. Each has its own hierarchical importance. All biodiversity components are interlinked and acting at any one level and have impact on other level of hierarchy, and have continuity amongst the different components from genes to ecosystems.

Besides its ecological and intrinsic value, biodiversity represents a considerable socio-economic and monetary asset as well. Human society depends on biological resources and their diversity, and the ecosystems that sustain them to provide essential goods and services. McNeely *et al*, (1990) classified the values of biodiversity into three categories. Productive use value: fuel wood, timber, fish, animal skins, musks, fooder, fruits, cereals, and medicinal plants come under this category. Consumptive use value: non-timber forest products such as soft broom grass and canefall. Indirect use value: prevention of soil erosion, maintenance of ecological balance, etc.

Today's biodiversity is a product of over 3.5 billion years of evolution, involving speciation, migration, extinction and more recently human influence. In recent times, a significant number of species are being lost much faster than the natural rate of extinction, due to increased human population and activities. A tremendous loss of genetic diversity have been noticed during the last hundred years. Many more species are on the verge of extinction. Inspite of extensive reserves of biological resources, India's biodiversity is at a higher risk of extinction. This is due to high degree of endamism. Therefore, protecting India's biodiversity is not only a national but a global concern. India occupies only 2.4 per cent of the world's land area but it shares 8 per cent world's biodiversity. Out of the total number of species (Khoshoo, 1995a) estimated to be 1.6 million (World Conservation Monitoring Centre, 1992) 1,26,188 have been described from India. The animal species groups which are most familiar with flowering plants (angiosperms) are mammals, fishes, birds, reptiles and amphibians constitutes 17.3 per cent of the total whereas, nearly 60 per cent of Inidia's bio-wealth is contribution of fungi and insects (Khoshoo, 1995b).

Indian agro-biodiversity is quite impressive. India ranks seventh in the world as far as the number of species contributed to agriculture and animal husbandry is concerned. Sustainable agriculture is an important component of overall sustainable development particularly for countries such as India where agriculture provides the livelihood for the three fourth of its population. Kumar (1998) estimated that by 2020 India will need 294 million tonnes of food grains *i.e.* 82 mt (million tonnes) more than that in 2001-02. This calls for producing 29 mt. more rice, 31 mt more wheat, 7 mt more coarse grains and 15 mt more pulses (beans) from the same or even lesser cultivated area. The yield of these crops have to be increased by 22 to 41 per cent in cereals and 110 per cent in pulses over that in 2001-02, which is a challenge to both agronomists and breeders. The environment is plagued with different kinds of pollutants. Continuous imbalanced use of fertilizers and indiscriminate use of pesticides on crops and soil along with organic wastes, including domestic and industrial sewage sludge and food processing wastes, cause serious environmental pollution (Mukhopadhay *et al*, 2005). Nevertheless caution needs to be exercised and agricultural practices that reduce the pollution of the environment need to be developed and practiced. In present study, the insect group selected is dragonflies (Order: Odonata) which acts as biocontrol agents of insect pests in aquatic and terrestrial ecosystems will solve the above pollution problem by reducing the risk of pesticides in environment.

HISTORICAL REVIEW OF THE PREVIOUS WORKS

From India Fabricius (1777, 1793 and 1798) and Rambur (1842) described several species mentioning their type locality, as "*Indes orientalis*" which do not clearly indicate, any specific locality. Ed de Selys Longchamps described several Indian species from localities belonging to Meghalaya. In 1853, Hagen and Selys described *Echo margarita* from a collection, which contained a specimen from Cherrapunjee in Meghalaya. Selys also described several species from Meghalaya namely *Philoganga montana* (as *Anisoneur montana*) (1959), *Gomphus personatus* (1873), *Idionyx optata* and *Hemicordulia asiatica* (1878), *Euphea orchracea brunnea* (as *Euphea brunnea*), *Bayadera hyalina; Echo margarita tripartita*, (*Citing tripartita* as a race), *Matrona basilaris nigripectus; Rhinocypha ignipennis, R. immaculata, R. spuria* and *Vestalaria smaragdina* (as *Vestalis smaragdina*) (1879), *Sympetrum orientale* (as *Diplax orientale*) (1883), *Sympetrum hypomelas* (as *Diplax hypomelas*) (1884) and *Etattoneura atkinsoni* (as *Disparoneura atkinsoni*) (1886). From Khasia hills Selys (1891) recorded *Aciagrion approximas* (Selys), *Orthetrum triangulare triangulare* (Selys) (as *Libella triangularia*) and *Trithemis festiva* Brauer. Later, McLachian (1896) described *Gynacantha khasiaca* from Khasi hills. Martin (1909) described *Aeshna petalura* and *Austroaeschna intersedens* and Ris (1916) described the subspecies *Neurothemis intermedia atlanta* from Khasi hills. Ris (1909-1919, 1912) confirmed the existence of some Odonate species earlier recorded from Meghalaya and also recorded a number of species, *viz. Bayadera indica* (Selys), *Crocothemis servilia servilia* (Drury), *Orthetrum glaucum* (Brauer), *O. luzonicum* (Brauer), *O. japonicum internum* McLachlan and *Trithemis aurora* (Burmeister) from the state. Laidlaw (1914, 1917a,b, 1919, 1921, 1922, 1932) described seven species and recorded three other species from Meghalaya these are *Coeliccia bimaculata* Laidlaw, *Indocnemis kempi* Liadlaw, *Acigrion tillyardi* Liadlaw, *Onychogomphus aureus* Laidlaw, *Anisogomphus orites* Laidlaw, *Coeliccia fraseri* Laidlaw, *C. vacca* Laidlaw, *Matrona basilaris basilaris* Selys, *Gynacantha hyalina* Selys and *Heliogomphus selysi* [as *H. nietneri* (Selys)]. Fraser (1919a, 1921c, 1922, 1924a, 1925a, 1926a,b, c, 1927a, 1929 a,c, 1930, 1935) contributed to 17 new species and one new race and recorded eight other species; these are *Rhinocypha quadrimaculata race hymihyalina* Fraser, *Pradasineura autumnalis* Fraser (as *Caconeura autumnalis*), *Indolestes indica* Fraser, *Pseudagrion spenci* Fraser, *Agriocnemis clauseni* Fraser, *Heliogomphus spirillus* Fraser (as *Leptogomphus spirillus*), *Megalogomphus bicornutus*) Fraser (as *Gomphus bicornutus*), *Merogomphus martini* Fraser (as *Platygomphus martini*), *Paragomphus echinogccipitalis* Fraser (as *Onychogomphus echinooccipitalis*), *Idionyx imbircata* Fraser, *I. intricata* Fraser, *Davidius malloryi* Fraser, *Anisogomphus caudalis* Fraser, *Anisopleura subplatystyla* Fraser, *Periaeschna nocturnalis* Fraser, *Petaliaes chna flatcheri* Fraser, *Dubitogomphus bidantatus* Fraser (as *Leptogomphus bidantatus*), *Periaeschna biguttata* (Fraser) (as *Cephalae schna bigutta*), *Palpopleura sexmaculata sexmaculata* (Fabricius), *Macromia moorei* Selys, *Ceriagrion olivaceum* Laidlaw, *Chlorogomphus atkinsoni* (Selys) (as *Orogomphus atkinsoni* Selys), *C. campioni* (Fraser) (as *O. campioni* Fraser), *Zygonyxi iris* Selys, *Euphaea ochracea* Selys (as *Allophae ochracea* Selys) and *Megalestes major* Selys. Needham (1932), Fraser and Laidlaw in their above mentioned contribution and Fraser (1918, 1919c, 1920c, 1922a, b, c,d, 1923d, 1924a, 1925b, c,d,e, 1912 b,c, 1928, 1929b, 1932, 1934) also confirmed the existence of several odonate species already known from Meghayala. Fraser (1933, 1934 and 1936) published accounts of Indian odonates. In these monographs Fraser gave description of the different taxonomic categories. In the fauna of Indian volumes Fraser (1933, 1934, 1936) recorded some odonate species and subspecies from Meghalaya, namely *Ceriagrion azureum* (Selys), *Caliphaea confusa* Selys, *Onchogomphus modestas* Selys (as *Nepogomphus modestus* (Selys)], *Chlorogomphus fraseri* St. Quentin, *Oligoaeschna martini* (Laidlaw), *Periaeschna magdalena* Martin, *Lyriothemis tricolor* Ris and *Zygonyx iris davina* Fraser.

Cowley (1936) described a new species from Khasi hills namely, *Bayodera kali* St. Quentin (1937) described *Anisopleura vallei* and the female of *Indocnemis kempi* Laidlaw from Cherrapunjee. Cowley (1937) discussed and illustrated the penile organs of some species of Chlorocyphidae occurring in Meghalaya. Fraser (1940) discussed and illustrated the penile organs of some species of *Gomphidae* occurring in Meghalaya. Lieftinck (1960) recorded *Anax guttatus* (Burmeister) from Meghayala on the basis of a female specimen captured from Khasi hills. Lieftinck (1968) described *Oligoaeschna decorata* and *O. khasiana* from Khasi hills. Asahina (1963), Bhasin (1963), Lieftinck (1948, 1960) and Vershney (1971) confirmed the existence of some Odonate species in the state, already recorded from the area. Kimmins (1966, 1968, 1969) designated lectotypes of some Odonate species and subspecies occurring in Meghalaya. Pinhey (1974) while revising the African species of *Agriocnemis* Selys redescribed *A. pygmaea* (Rumbur) and cited the differences between Shillong and Seychelles forms of this species. Lahari (1975) discussed the behaviour of *Bayadera hyalina* Selys in Shillong region during the rains. Lahiri (1976) described *Calicnemia mukherjeei* from Shillong. Lieftinck (1977) described *Somatochlora deviesi* from Khasi hills. Thus, till the present work, 82 Odonate species and sub species under 49 genera belonging to 14 families were known from Meghalaya.

Prasad and Varshany (1988) published the Odonata of Bihar, India under which they described 63 species and sub-species of Bihar. They also contributed on generic distribution and zoogeography of Odonata of Bihar. They reported four endemic species from Bihar. Out of 63 species 13 species were newly described by them.

Prasad (1995) reported 22 species of Odonata belonging to 16 genera and 15 families for the first time from Goa. All these species agree fairly well with the description of Fraser (1933, 1934 and 1936). Asahima (1961) described larval forms of dragonflies from Darjiling. Asahima (1981) reviewed the Himalayan dragonfly genus *Cephalaeschna*. Singh and Prasad (1974, 1976) studied dragonflies of North West India. Similarly, Singh and Baijal (1954) and Singh *et al.* (1955) studied dragonflies of Himalayan region. Tyagi (1984) reported dragonflies from Chandigarh. Sahni (1964) made the survey of dragonflies of Nainital. Rao and Laheri (1982) studied Odonata of salient valley and New Amarbalom reserved forests. Ram *et al.* (1982) studied fauna of Calcutta. Ram *et al.* (1983) also studied Odonata from eastern Uttar Pradesh. Prasad and Ghosh (1984b) studied Odonata from Sikkim. In addition several other workers not listed in text but cited in bibliography have studied Indian Odonata. Joseph (1988) studied Odonata from Andhra Pradesh, India. Kumar (1990) studied Odonata of Vedanthangal Water Bird Sanctuary, Tamil Nadu. Lahiri (1991) studied the Odonata fauna of Chilka lake. Laidlaw (1915a) noted oriental dragonflies in the Indian Museum. Laidlaw (1916b, 1919, 1920, 1921, 1922a) studied Indian dragonflies. Laidlaw (1924) studied oriental dragonflies of the genus *Aciagrion*. Mani (1955) published a monomental work, Entomological Survey of the Himalayas Part IX, First annotated check list of Insects from the North-West (Punjab) Himalayas. Mitra (1975) studied fauna of Tripura. Prasad (1980) studied Odonata from Khasi Hills, Meghalaya. Prasad (1981) studied Odonata from Rajasthan. Asahima (1967) studied three Indian dragonfly species. Asahima (1981) studied the Himalayan dragonflies of the genus *Cephalaeschna* and its allies (Odonate, Aesnidae), Bhasin (1953) studied Odonata (In Roonwal, M.L. *et al.*, 1953 A systematic catalogue of the main identified collection at the FRI, Dehra Dun, part 9-21) of Dehra Dun. Dasgupta (1957) studied cytological aspects of Indian dragonflies. Fraser (1921c) recorded a list of dragonflies from Mahabaleshwar. Mitra (1983) published a list of Odonata from Calcutta.

Out of 6000 species reported from the world, 650 species belonging to 139 genera of 17 families have been reported from India (Kulkarni and Prasad, 2002). Recently, Prasad and Kulkarni (2001) reported 71 species from Nilgiri Biosphere reserve and its environs. Prasad and Kulkarni (2002) also reported additional 34 species from Kerala. From Western Ghats 138 species have been reported. Most of the studies are confined to Western Ghats of Kerala and very little attention is paid on the Western Ghats of Maharashtra region. Western Ghats is among the 18 hot spots of the World and needs conservation and protection of biodiversity including dragonflies. Therefore, attempts have been made on biodiversity of Western Ghats of Maharashtra region. In past Fraser (1933, 1934, 1936); Prasad (1995, 1996), Prasad and Varshney (1995), Prasad and Kulkarni (2001, 2002), Kulkarni and Prasad (2002), Sathe *et al.* (2005), Sathe and Shinde (2006) etc. have worked on biodiversity of Odonata from Western Ghats.

TAXONOMICAL CONSIDERATIONS

KEY TO THE SUBORDERS OF ORDER ODONATA

Distance between inner margins of eyes greater than own diameter in males interior and appendage paired and placed below anal opening. Fore and hind wings more or less similar in shape and venation ....Zygoptera.

Distance between inner margins of eyes always less than their own diameter in males interior and appendage single and placed above anal opening. Fore and hind wings different in shape and venation ....Anisoptera

Suborder Zygoptera

The suborder Zygoptera is characterised by head transversely elongated; middle lobe of labium fissured and subequal to lateral lobe; distance between inner margins of eyes greater than their own diameter; ocelli not set in vesicle, lying free in middle of vertex; occiput. trapezoidal; male genitalia with deeply cleft lamina, with anterior hamules well developed, posterior hamules inconspicuous and lobe elongated; both superior and inferior anal appendages in male paired and placed above and below anal opening respectively; female with fully developed ovipositor. Fore and hind wings similar in shape and venation; discoidal cell in the form of a quadrangle.

Distribution

Cosmopolitan.

KEY TO THE SUPERFAMILIES OF THE SUBORDER ZYGOPTERA

1. More than 2 antenodal cross veins present; postnodales not in alignment with veins beneath...................Calopterygoidea
   only 2 antenodal cross veins present; postnodals in strict alignment with cross veins beneath...2
2. Origin of IR_3 and R_{4+5} generally more near nodus than or even beyond level of nodus males with anterior hamules subquadrate..*Coenagrionoidea*

Origin of IR_3 and R_{4+5} generally more than near are more than nodus males with anterior hamules elongated....................................*Lestidoidea*

Superfamily CALOPTERYGOIDEA

The superfamily shows following features: Medium to large sized insects; hind margin of posterior lobe of prothroax rounded, trapezoidal, or shallowly tripertite; prothorax usually with a boss on either side, males with anterior hamules quadrate. Wings usually petiolated, sometimes not petiolated; more than two (usually more than 5) antenodal cross veins present; postnodals not in strict alignment with cross veins beneath; IR_3 and R_{4+5} usually beginning nearer than nodus; a number of intercalated sectors present, at least between branches of Rs and MA.

Distribution

Virtually cosmopolitan.

KEY TO THE FAMILIES OF THE SUPERFAMILY CALOPTERYGOIDEA

1. Two primary antenodal cross veins easily distinguishable from the secondaries.......................2
   Two primary antenodal cross veins not distinguishable from the secondaries.................................3
2. Petiolation of wing ending opposite to or slightly proximal to the level of erc..*Amphipterygidae*
   Petiolation of wing ending for proximal to the level of arc...*Chlorocyphidae*
3. 1st lateral suture of synthorax incomplete and not traceable up to the spiracle.....................*Euphaeidae*
   1st lateral suture of synthorax complete and well developed, traceable even beyond spiracle..*Calopterygidae*

Family AMPHIPTERYGIDAE

Diagnostic characters: Large in size; ground colour without metallic lusture. Wings hyaline; petiolation ending, at or slightly proximal to the level of arc; more than two antenodal cross veins present; primary anternodals easily distinguishable, other antenodals present either only in costal space or in both costal and subcostal space and then these not coinciding; discoidal cells short and broad or long and narrow, entire or transversed by cross veins; base of discoidal cell connected to radius by arc; arc slightly bent, situated in line with distal antenodal cross vein; sectors of arc arising from above the middle of these being either separated at origin or arising from a common point or even from a common stalk; IR_3 arising closer to arc or midway between arc and nodus where it is close or widely spaced with $R_{4+5.}$

The family is distributed in India, China, Burma, Thailand, Malaysia, Indonesia, Australia, Africa and South Amercia.

Suborder ANISOPTERA

Diagnostic Characters

Head compact, more or less globular; labium with middle lobe usually smaller than lateral lobes and with or without a median fissure; inner margin of eyes never separated by a space greater than their own diameter; male genitalia variable, lamina usually arched, both hamules or only the posterior one well developed; paired superior and single inferior anal appendage present in males, all placed above anal opening; ovipositor variable in female, either fully developed or aborted. Fore and hind wing dissimilar in venation and outline, anal field of hind wing broader than that of forewing; usually more than 5 antenodal cross veins present in all wings; discoidal cell differentiated into a triangle and a hypertriangle.

KEY TO THE SUPERFAMILIES OF THE SUBORDER ANISOPTERA

1. Labial mask of nymphs of primitive
   zygopterous type, flattened and without setae;
   lateral lobes narrow, with a long robust
   movable hook; gizzard with 4-8 folds,
   each with numerous small teeth............................*Aeshnoidea*

Labial mask of nymph broad and deeply concave or cupped and with numerous setae; lateral lobes broad, their apposed borders being more or less deeply incised, crenate or serrate and often bordered with tuft of setae; gizzard with 4 folds, each a robust tooth...2

2. Adults with costal and subcostal cross veins not coinciding; inner margin of eyes in adults very slightly separated or meeting only at a point; adult males with anterior and posterior hamules of genitalia well developed and females without ovipositor of only with pseudovipositor......................................*Cordulegasteroidea*
3. Adults with costal and subcostal antenodal cross veins coinciding inner margin of eyes in adults broadly contiguous adults males with obsolete anterior hamules of genitalia and females with ovipositor usually inconspicuous..*Libelluloidea*

Superfamily AESHNOIDEA

This superfamily shows following features:

Head nearly globular; inner margins of eyes contiguous or well separated; vesicle not well differentiated; occiput large or small, trapezoidal or triangular; male genitalia with well developed hamules; ovipositor present or absent. Costal and subcostal antenodal cross veins not coinciding; two primary antenodal cross veins usually well developed. This super family is distributed throughout the world.

KEY TO THE FAMILIES OF THE SUPERFAMILY AESHNOIDEA

1. Inner margins of eyes well separated; occipital plate large and trapezoidal; female without ovipositor....................................*Gomphidae*
2. Inner margins of eyes broadly contiguous on vertex; occipital plate small and triangular; female with well-developed ovipositor...*Aeshnidae*

Family GOMPHIDAE

Diagnostic Characters

Head subglobular; labium with middle lobe lacking median incision, broader than lateral lobes; inner margins of eyes well separated; occiput large, transversely elongate and trapezoidal; male genitalia not covered by 2nd abdominal tergite; ovipositor absent; vulver scale usually present, subtrigone well differentiated, it and hypertrigone entire or transversed by cross veins; discoidall cell entire or traversed by cross veins, similar or dissimilar in shape in fore and hind wings; usually 1-4 cross veins in cubital space and 2-8 cross veins between R_3 and MA in hindwing; forking of R_3 symmetrical or asymmetrical; median space entire; anal loop rudimentary or absent.

Distribution

Cosmopolitan

MORPHOLOGICAL CONSIDERATION

Morphological details of dragonfly are shown in Figures 1–9.

HEAD (Figure 1)

Head is composed mainly of two large compound eyes which are fused broadly across the middle line, in most Anisoptera and merely meet at a point in the more primitive Anisoptera and are slightly or widely separated in the Zygoptera. There are three tiny ocelli situated between and infront of the former or grouped round a small eminence known as the vesicle. The antennae (Figure 2) are

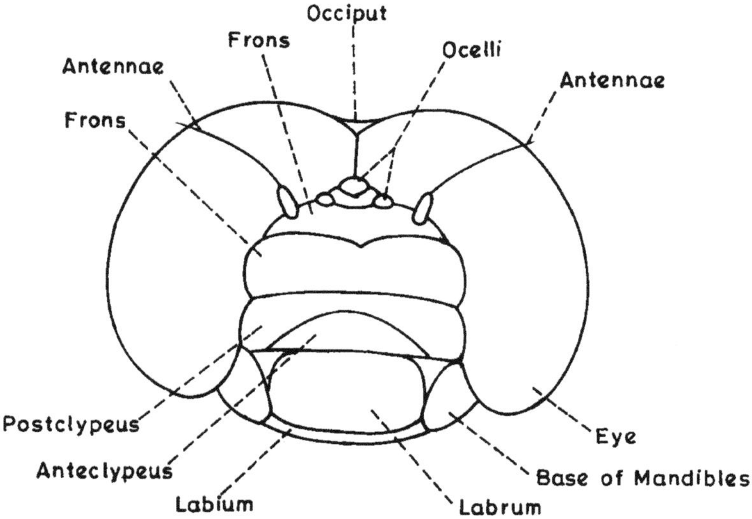

Figure 1: Head of an Anisopterous Dragonfly Seen from the Front

very short and inconspicuous, filiform, composed of four to seven segments. The mouth parts are biting type. The mandibles are with strong incisor and molar teeth. The maxillae are with simple unjointed jap and robustly toothed internal lobe. The labrum (Figure 1) is upper lip of mouth. The labium is short and very broad, made up of median and two lateral lobes. The former cleft in the zygoptera is more archaic types, the latter smaller than the median lobe in the Zygoptera, larger in the Anisoptera and higher types, and made up of two segments, a basal and a large movable hook.

THORAX (Figure 3)

Thorax is composed of a small prothorax which forms a neck, and a larger mass the synthorax formed from the fusion of meso and metathorax. With the help of the prothorax, the insect is able to move its head freely in all directions mainly by the aid of its fore legs, which are used to push the head into various positions. The prothorax consists of an anterior lobe, collar-like consists of an anterior lobe, collar-like and narrow, a middle lobe, tumid and forming the greater part of the structure and lastly, a posterior lobe important for the purposes of classification, as its shape differs not only in the genera, but also in the species of individual genera; the posterior lobe is often armed with hooks or spines on its hinder border in the female, more rarely in the male also. The synthorax is a very oblique so that the anterior surface comes to be the dorsum, carrying back the wings and thrusting the legs forward beneath the head.

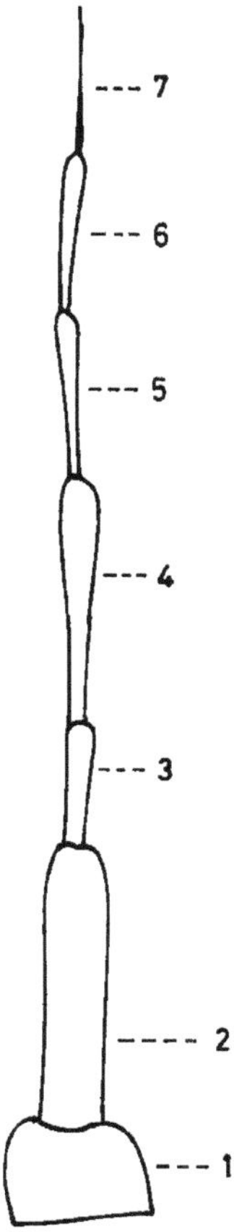

Figure 2: Antenna of Dragonfly
1: Scape; 2: Pedicel;
3–7: Flagellum

LEGS (Figure 4)

Legs are not used for walking but are formed for clinging and for catching prey for this latter purpose their legs are bunched together to form an open basket. The long spines are situated on the femora and tibia. Coxa is short and robust; trochanters slender, formed of two segments; tibia in some genera keeled, in others much dilated; tarsi made up of three segments, the terminal one ending in a pair of claws which usually bear a minute spine near the end.

WINGS (Figures 5 and 6)

During rest the wings are held vertically over the thorax and abdomen as in the zygoptera or opened widely and horizontally as in Philoganga and the Anisoptera. In some genera, such as *Leastes*, the wings are held half open during rest. The wings of dragonflies are membranous hyaline and with strong veins. The wings are partly with hairs or scales, or uncoloured or without hairs or scales but has numerous fine spines on the under surface of the supporting ribs or nervures of the wings.

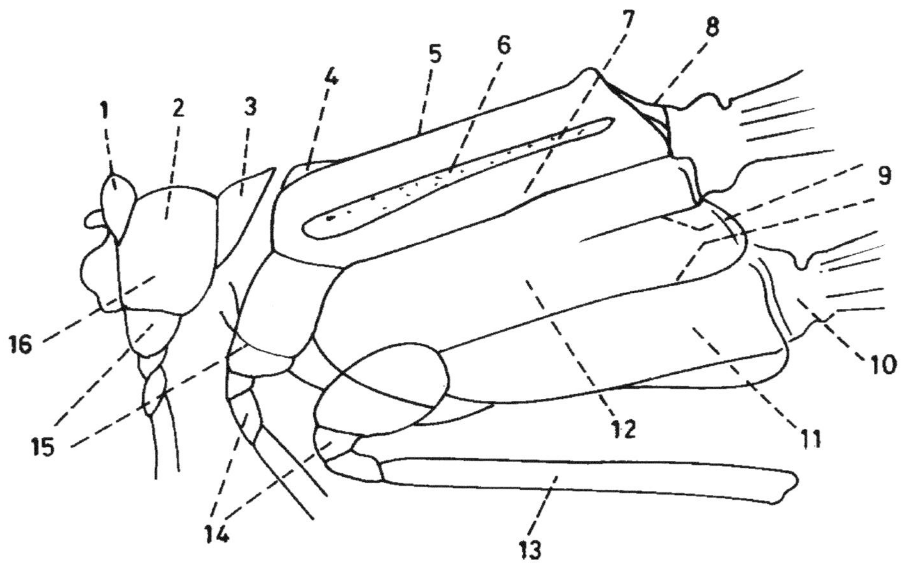

Figure 3: Prothorax and Synthorax of Dragonfly

1: Anterior lobe of prothorax; 2: Middle lobe of prothorax; 3: Posterior lobe of prothorax; 4: Mesothorasic triangle; 5: Middorsal cranial suture of ridge; 6: Ante humeral coloured striple 7: Humeral suture; 8: Ante-alar-sinus; 9: Anterior lateral suture; 10: Wing bases; 11: Metepimeron; 12: Mesepimeron; 13: Femur; 14: Trochanter 15: Coxa; 16: Prothorax

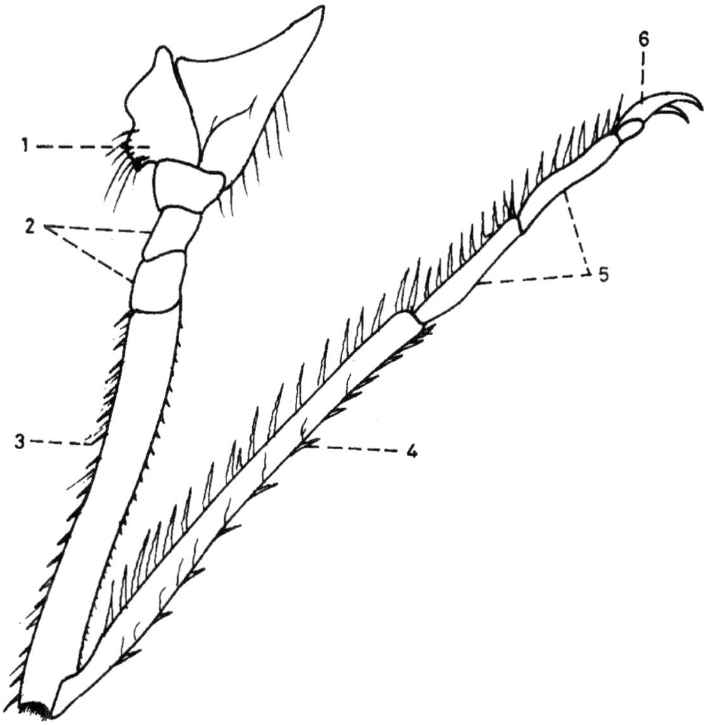

Figure 4: Leg of Dragonfly (Anisoptera)

1: Coxa; 2: Trochanter; 3: Femur; 4: Tibia; 5: Tarsus; 6: Claw

The venation is highly specialized. Several systems of notation are in vogue- the old Solysian system, which is more a nomenclature than a notation. The Comstock–Needham system is still employed by several specialists in the order. The revised and more modern Tillyard notation, which seeks to interpret the homologies of the veins and bring their notation into line with that of other orders of insects have been employed in present study for avoiding confusion. However, a comparative tabular form with the other two systems is given below (Table 1).

The classification of dragonflies have been largely depended upon the variations of structure of the wings and hence necessary to recognize certain parts and nervures (veins or ribs) in these organs. The important parts of the wings (Figures 5 and 6) are:

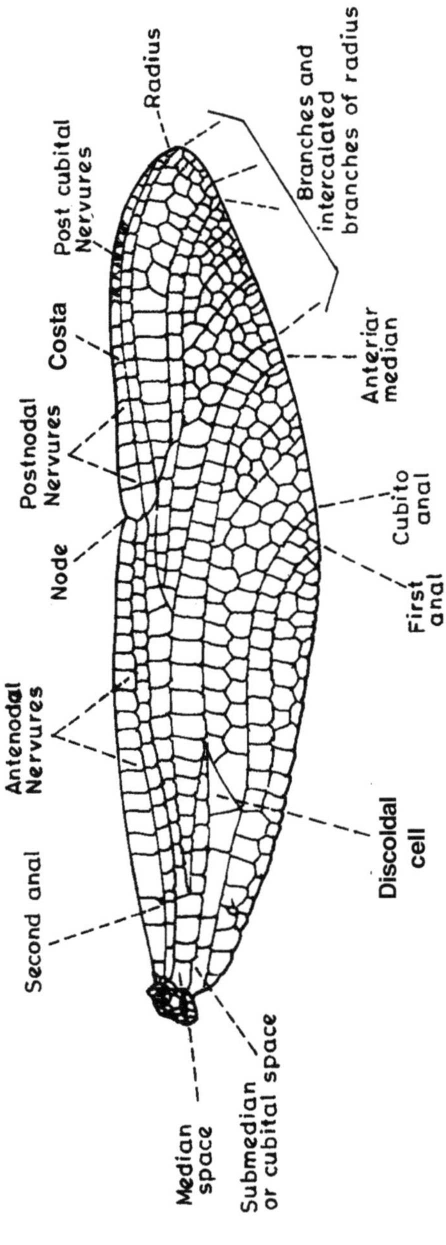

Figure 5: Fore Wing of Anisopterous Dragonfly

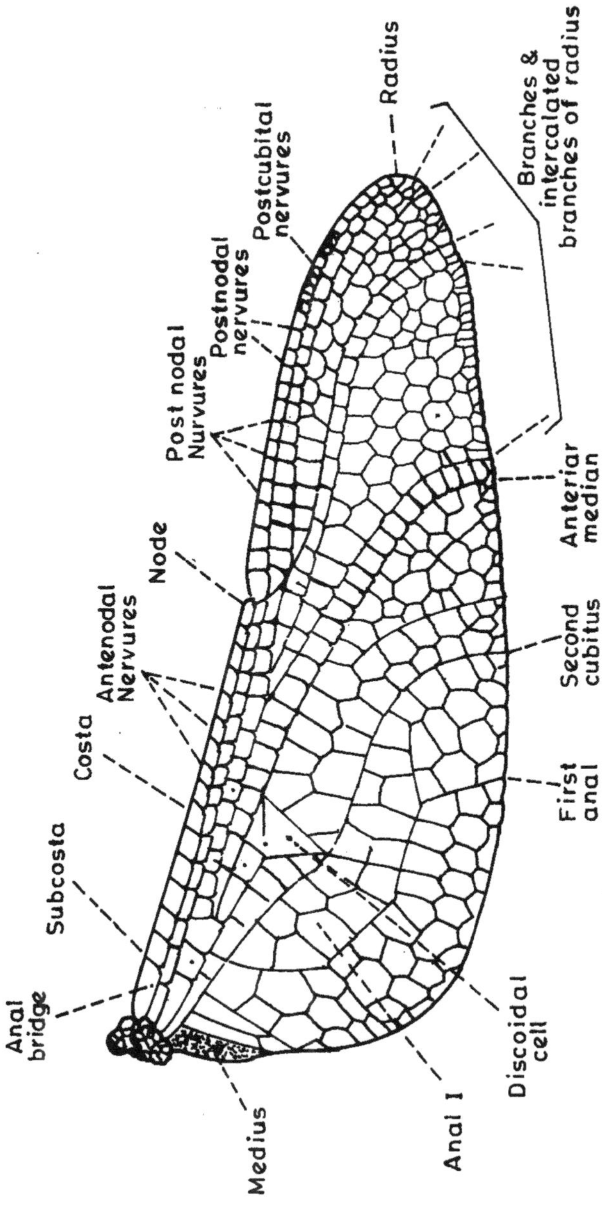

Figure 6: Hind Wing of Anisopterous Dragonfly

The Costa (C)

Anterior border of wing from base to apex.

The Node (N)

An artificial joint in the costa situated variably at or proximal to it's middle.

Table 1: Systems of Notation in Odonata

	Tillyard's	*Comstock Needham's*	*Solysian*
Costa	C	C	Costal nervure
Subcosta	Sc	Sc	Subcostal nervure
Radius median	R+M	R+M	Median nervure
Radius	Ri	Ri	Median nervure
Arculus vein	R_3+m	M	Arc
Radial sector	RS	Mi + iii	Sector of arc
	Rii	Mi	Principal sector
	IRii	Mia	Postnodal sector
Branches and	Riii	Mii	Nodal sector
Intercalated branches	IRiii	$R_3(M_3)$	Subnodal sector
of radius	Riv + V	Miii	Median sector
Anterior median	MA	Miv	Inferior sector of arc
Posterior median	(Absent in the odonata)		
First cubitus	Cui (Absent in the odonata)		
Second cubitus	Cuii	Cui	Superior sector of triangle
First anal	IA	Cuii	Inferior sector of triangle
Cubito anal	Cuii+IA	Cu	Submedian nervure
Second anal	A'	A	Postcostal nervure

Pterostigma

A thickened chitinized variably shaped cell situated on the costal margin near the apices of the wings. It may be absent in one or other wing or in one of the sexes, and may be placed, or not, at it's proximal end.

The Base

The side nearest the body of the insect. The wings are an

elongated triangle, the third side being known as the hind or posterior margin.

Spaces

Certain areas of the wing near the base have received names, and are noted in the diagram.

Nervures

These are the ribs of scaffolding on which the membrane is built up and comprise the costa, subcosta, a many branched radius, median cubital and anal nervures.

Discoidal Cell (DC)

Near the base of each wing will be found a triangular or quadrilateral cell which acts as a key stone from which other nervures appear to radiate. This cell is triangular in the *Anisoptera* and made up of two cells known as the trigone of triangle and the hypertrigone or hypertangle, but is a single quadrilateral cell in the *Zygoptera* where it is known as the quadrilateral. It is here called the discoidal cell, as it functions similarly to that space found in the wings of Lepidoptera.

Subnode (Sn)

The oblique nervure descending from the node.

Antenodal Nervure (An)

Antecubital nervures and postnodal nervures (Pn) postcubital nervures: These are nervures lying respectively between the costa and subcosta, and costa and radius on the proximal and distal sides of the node.

Median Space (Ms)

Some times called the basal space. It lies proximal to the arc, between it and the base of wing, and may be traversed by the nervures or entire, a distinction of generic value in the Zygoptera.

Submedian or Cubital Space (Cs)

Lies beneath and parallel to the median space between the base of the wing and discoidal cell.

Anal Bridge (Ab)

A short nervure running parallel to the hinder border of the wing and passing below the discoidal cell, variable in the genera of the Zygoptera complete or incomplete, usually arising from the hinder border of the wing at or proximal to the level of the nervure. Ac and extending out of the medio-anal link or underside of discoidal cell.

Anal Crossing (AC)

A short nervure situated at the base of the wing extending from Cuii + IA to the anal bridge or hinder border of the wing where the neuration is at all dense. This nervure will be indistinguishable from the general neuration.

ABDOMEN (Figures 6a, 7, 8 and 9)

The abdomen is ten segmented. In majority of the Zygoptera the abdomen is elongated and cylindrical and less than other suborders in length. The abdomen may be short, broad, flattened or tumid in parts, constricted or fujiform. The anal appendages are attached to the last segment.

Male Genitalia

Situated on the ventral surface of segment 2 and comprising the lamina, a hook like structure closing in the genital sac nearest the thorax; the hamules or hooks are used for copulating with the female. An anterior and posterior pair being usually present infinite in shape and variety. The penis an intricate organ varying greatly in the families, genera, and even in the species. It takes the form of a chitinized stem with a membranous apex which is bent strongly or folded back over the stem and furnished or not, with long and curling branches. The lobe, a small flask-shaped receptacle at the apical border of the 2nd segment, in which the apex of the penis is tucked away when not in use and which is also employed as a receptacle for the sperm.

The primitive penis is absent, but there is a gonopore at the junction of the 9th and 10th segments, from which the spermatozoa are at first passed into the lobe on segment 2 by the insect curling its abdomen underneath until the two segments are in juxtaposition, copulation then takes place with the female by means of the functional penis.

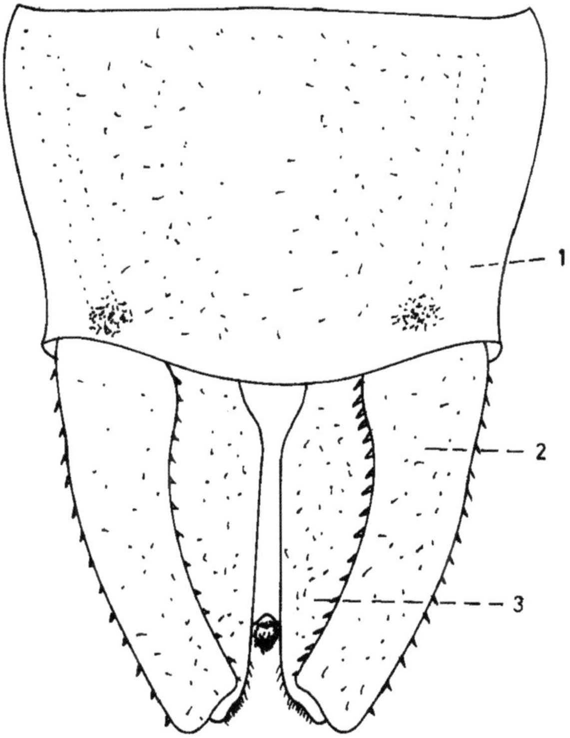

Figure 6a: Male Anal Appendages of Dragonfly in Dorsal View
1: 10th abdoinal segment; 2: Superior anal appendages; 3: Inferior anal appendages

Female Genitalia

The organs of female consist in all the Zygoptera and some of the Anisoptera of a robust ovipositor on the under side of segment 9 enclosed by a pair of vulvar scales or plates furnished with style which are probably tactile organs.

Anal Appendages (Figures 6a, 7, 8 and 9)

The Anisoptera possess a pair of superior and a single inferior as anal appendages but the zygoptera have in the male sex both paired superior and inferior appendages. These organs are employed in seizing the female by the head or prothorax prior to copulation

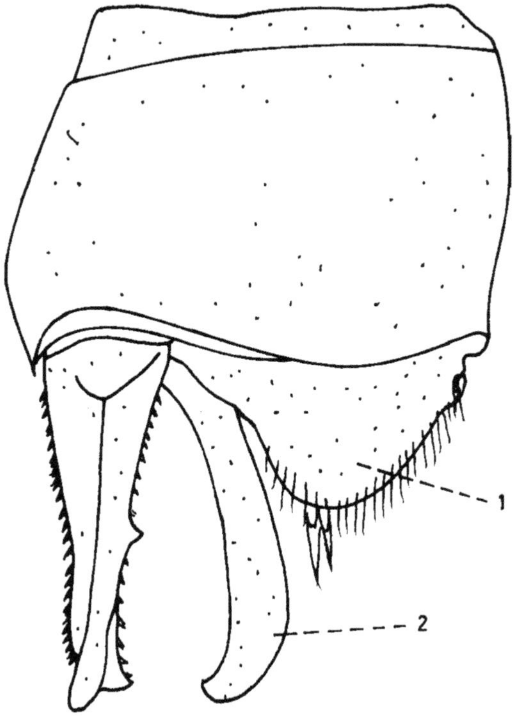

Figure 7: Male Anal Appendages of Dragonfly in Right Lateral View

1: Paraproct; 2: Inferior anal appendages

and arc of infinitely varied design, length and shape, furnishing a facinating study of the order whilst often of generic value, they are more useful as a specific character.

GENUS *MESOGOMPHUS* FORSTER

The genus *Mesogomphus* is raised by Forster in 1906. This genus is distributed in trophical Africa, Madagaster, India, Myanmar, Sri Lanka, Malaysia, Java and Celebes. From India five species have been reported. Species of this genus breed in open rocky streams, the males haunting shallow runnels where the water flows swiftly over a clean sandy or pebbly bottom, or they may be found setting on sandy beaches beside streams, including in frequent rapid flights

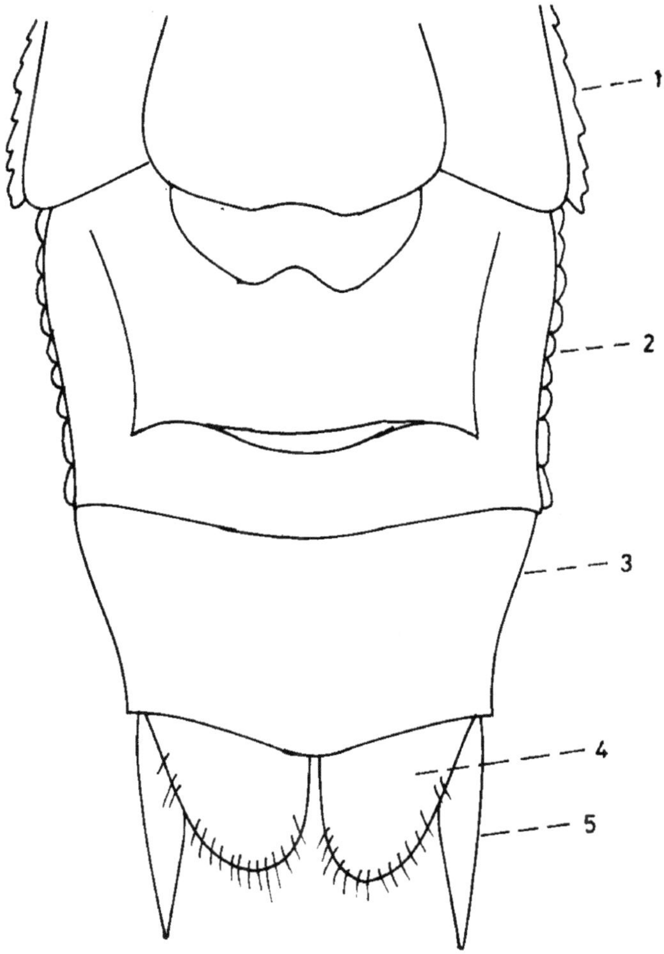

Figure 8: End Segments of Dragonfly Abdomen including Appendages Showing Female Genital Appendages in Dorsal View

1,2,3: Abdominal segments; 4: Epiproct; 5: Anal appendages

up and down stream. The larvae resemble those of *Burmagomphus* and *Onchogomphus* and have similar habits. The genus is closely related to *Onychogomphus,* from which it is distinguished by the dilated and winged lateral borders of segments 8 and 9 as well by

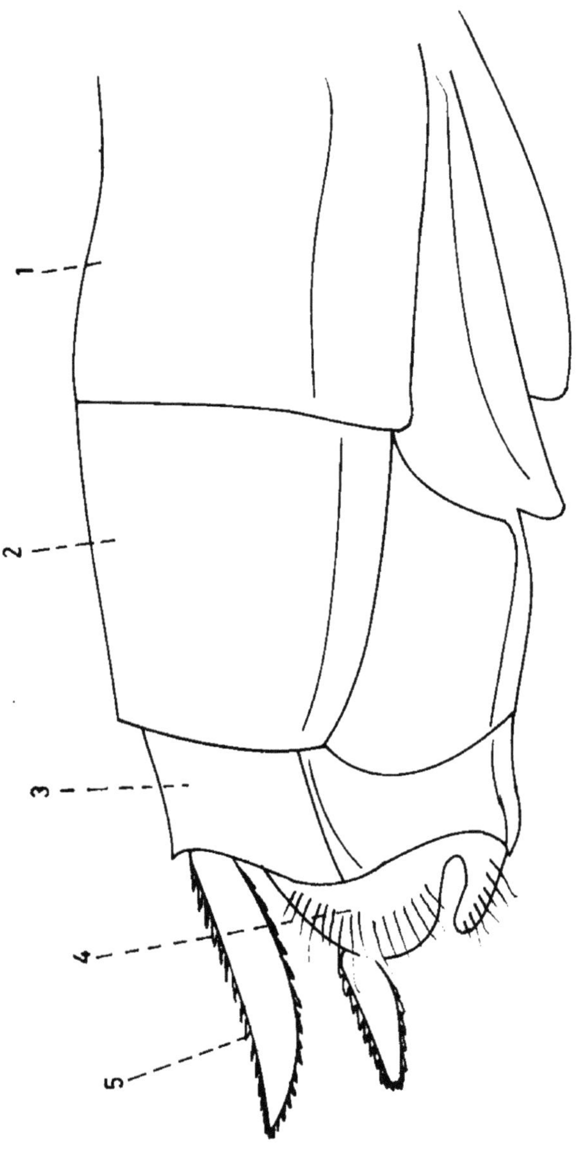

Figure 9: End Segments of Dragonfly Abdomen including Anal Appendages Showing Female Genitalia in Right Lateral View

1,2,3: Abdominal segments; 4: Epiproct; 5: Anal appendages

the absence of an anal loop in the hind-wing. The larvae burrow in sand and are stream dwellers.

This genus show following characters

1. Size medium, colour for the most part sandy yellow marked with shades of brown and black.
2. Head moderately large, triangular.
3. Frons angulated.
4. Occiput simple, usually slightly and shallowly concave.
5. Wings: reticulation close, tornus angulated and base of hind-wing moderately excavated; membrane very narrow, almost obsolete; anal triangle 4-celled; are situated midway between the first and second antenodal nervures: only 2 transverse nervures between the sectors of arc from arc to bifurcation of RS in the fore wings.
6. Pterostigma rather long, expanded at its middle, well braced, slightly longer than one third the distance from node to proximal end of pterostigma.
7. Subtrigones and hypertrigones entire in all wings.
8. Legs short, hind femora extending only to posterior margin of thorax and furnished with a dense group of short spines on proximal half of flexor surface which become more or less arranged into two rows at distal end of femur; tibial spines moderately short and closely set.
9. Abdomen of male tumid at base, narrow and cylindrical from segment 3 to base of segment 7 from which point the abdomen is again dilated, especially at segments 8 and 9 which bear broad lateral wing like projections very similar to those found in species of the genus *Ictinus*.
10. Abdomen of female more or less cylindrical throughout, segments 8 and 9 without lateral dilatations.
11. Anal appendages; superiors nearly double the length of segment 10, tapering to apex, the terminal half curled regularly downwards and very closely apposed; inferior less than half the length of superiors, strongly curled in a downward and then an upward direction, bifid nearly to base, the two branches closely apposed like the superiors.

Mesogomphus Forster, Wiesbaden Jahr, ver, Natk. vol. lix, p. 323, (1906): Ris, Ann. S. Afr. Mus. Vol. xviii, p. 343 (1920); Fraser, J. Bombay Nat. Hist Soc. Lond. Vol. lxxviii, p. 192 (1930); Needham, Rec. Ind. Mus. vol., xxxiv, pp. 217, 218, 221 (1932).

MESOGOMPHUS INDICA SP. NOV.

MALE (Figures 10, 11)

Body 45.00 mm long excluding anal appendages; head 3.00 mm long, thorax 11.00 mm long, fore wing 26.00 mm long, hind wing 24.00 mm long, abdomen 31.00 mm long, yellow with black patches on dorsal side; anal appendages 2.70 mm long, reddish brown with black tip.

HEAD

3.00 long, 6.00 mm broad, roughly triangular; occiput brown with hairs, compound eyes brown with black and red patches; occular space 3.00 mm; three ocelli in triangle, black with basally faint yellow ring, ocellar space 0.26 mm, interocellar space 1.80 mm, frons whitish with black transverse stripe on front side; postclypeus, anteclypeus, white; labrum whitish; mandible brown, mandible bases yellow; labium whitish with mid lobe black.

Antenna

1.22 mm long, 0.26 mm broad (width of scape 0.26 mm), 7 segmented; scape 0.10 mm long, 0.26 mm broad, black; pedicel 0.26 mm long, 0.22 mm broad, black. Flagellum: 5 segmented 0.86 mm long, 0.6 mm broad, brown, 1st segment 0.20 mm long, 0.06 mm broad; 2nd segment 0.12 mm long, 0.04 mm broad; 3rd segment 0.12 mm long, 0.022 mm broad; 4th segment 0.10 mm long, 0.014 mm broad; 5th segment 0.32 mm long, 0.009 mm broad.

Flagellar Formula

L/W; ½ = 3.33/3; $^{2/2}$ = 3/3; $^{3/2}$ = 5.45/3; $^{4/2}$ = 7.14/3; $^{5/2}$ = 35.55/3; A = 3.62.

THORAX

11.00 mm long, 5.00 mm broad, with yellow black and brown stripes on vetrolaterally. Prothorax 5.50 mm long, 5.00 mm broad, 3 lobed, with yellow and brown stripes on ventral and lateral side;

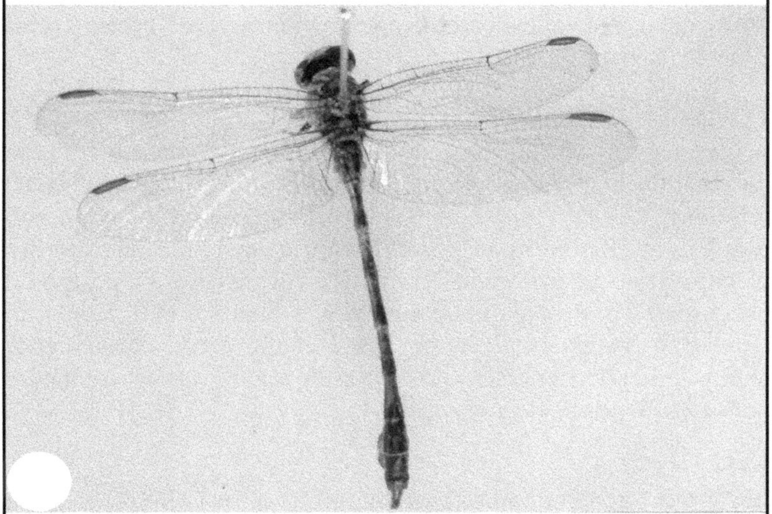

Figure 10: ***Mesogomphus indica*** **sp.nov.; Male**

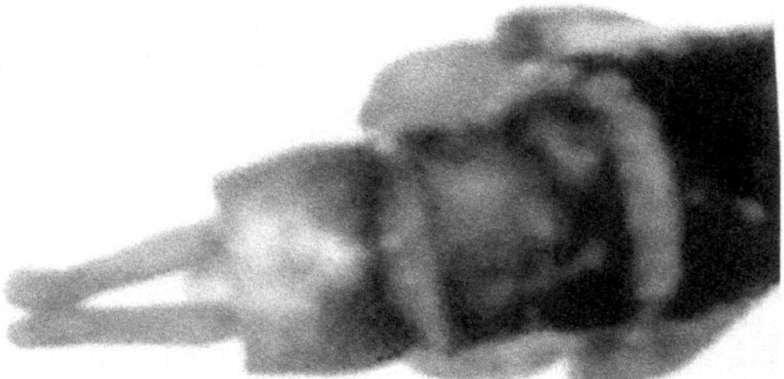

Figure 11: ***Mesogomphus indica:*** **Anal Appendages; Male**

anterior lobe 0.9 mm long, black with dense hairs; middle lobe 4.20 mm long, 5.00 mm broad with mid dorsal side brown and at lateral side two greenish and two black stripes and one small brown plate on mid dorsal at posterior region and one yellow transverse ring on anterior region; posterior lobe 0.3 mm long, 5.00 mm broad, robust with dorsal side yellow patches and on ventral side 3 greenish and 3 blackish stripes.

WINGS (Figure 10)

Wings hyaline, wing apices black and pointed, close reticulation, black venations, wing bases pointed. Fore wing: 26.00 mm long, 7.00 mm broad, 56.00 mm wing span; pterostigma 3.40 mm long, 0.70 mm broad, costal border yellow and inner border black and middle surface yellow; antenodal nervures 12, postnodal nervures 9. Hind wing: 24.00 mm long, 8.00 mm broad, 52.00 mm wing span, pterostigma 2.90 mm long, 0.70 mm broad, costal border yellow, inner border black and on middle region yellow; antenodal nervures 11; postnodal nervures 8.

LEG

Hind leg 12.50 mm long, 1.20 mm broad (width of coxa 1.20 mm); coxa 0.90 mm long, 1.20 mm broad, yellowish with reddish patch; trochanter 2 segmented, 1.70 mm long, 0.56 mm broad, 1st segment 0.70 mm long, 0.56 mm broad, yellow with inner side black; 2nd segment 1.00 mm long, 0.56 mm broad, 0.20 mm part of trochanter overlaps on coxa, yellow with inner side black and 4 small black spines on inner side; femora 4.30 mm long, 0.76 mm broad, yellow on anterior side and on posterior side black patch with many small, black, blunt spines on inner side; tibia 2.80 mm long, 0.32 mm broad, black with posterior side yellow patch and 11 black thick spines on inner side; tarsus 3 segmented 1.80 mm long, 0.26 mm broad, black; 1st segment 0.80 mm long, 0.24 mm broad with 5 black thick spines on inner side, 2nd segment 0.40 mm long, 0.26 mm broad with 3 spines on inner side, 3rd segment 0.60 mm long, 0.26 mm broad with 4 spines on inner side; claw 0.70 mm long, 0.16 mm broad, reddish with 2 spines.

ABDOMEN

31.00 mm long, 3 mm broad, yellow with black patches; 1st segment yellow with apically black; 2nd segment broad,with two black spots on dorsolateral side; 3, 4, 5, 6 and 7 segment reddish brown with black patches on basal region; 8th segment blackish brown, 9th segment reddish brown with black patches on dorsal side, 10th segment small, blackish brown with two black spots on dorsolateral side; segment 9th and 10th with two reddish flaps on ventrolater side. Anal appendages (Figure 11): Reddish brown, 2.70 mm long, 0.50 mm broad; superior anal appendages 2.70 mm long, 0.50 mm broad, basally reddish brown with very small black tip; inferior 170 mm long, 50 mm broad, reddish brown, cylindrical.

COLOUR

Brown: Occiput; compound eyes.

Black: Ocelli, tarsus.

Whitish: Frons, postclypeus, anteclypeus, labium.

Reddish brown: Anal appendages.

Yellow: Abdomen.

Yellowish: Coxa, trochanter.

PREY RECORD: Midgefly *Contariuia* sp.,

Mosquitoes *Culex* sp.

HOLOTYPE: Male, India, Maharashtra, Coll. 10-X-2004; Kamargaon, Satara district, M.S., Shinde, K.P. antenna, leg on slide labelled as above, other parts with pined form, labelled as above.

PARATYPE: Male 1, Coll. 21-XI-2004; same data as above.

DISTRIBUTIONAL RECORD/OBSERVATIONS

Male 18, female 1. Kargaon ♂1, 14-XI-2004; Khirkhindi ♂1, 19-XII-2004; Sondari ♂1 ♀1, 26-XII-2004; Rohine ♂4, 13-II-2005; Tapola ♂2, 10-IV-2005; Sondari ♂2, 15-V-2005; Munawale ♂3, 22-V-2005; Navaja ♂3, 11-IX-2005; Nisare ♂1, 5-II-2006.

DISCUSSION

This species runs close to *Mesogomphus frontalis* (Selys) by following characters

1. Hind femora yellow.
2. Occiput brown.
3. Abdomen length between 30 mm to 39 mm.

However, it differs from the above species by having following characters:

1. Frons whitish.
2. Labrum whitish.

3. Anal appendages reddish brown.
4. Flagellar formula: L/W; $^{1/2}$ = 3.33/3; $^{2/2}$ = 3/3; $^{3/2}$ = 5.45/3; $^{4/2}$ = 7.14/3; $^{5/2}$ = 35.55/3; A = 3.62.
5. Thorax black and brown stripes on ventrolaterally.
6. Fore wing: Pterostigma yellow with black border not brown with black.
7. Hind wing: Pterostigma yellow with black border.
8. In fore wing: antenodal nervures 12, post nodal nervures 9.
9. In hind wing, antenodal nervures 11, post nodal nervures 8.
10. Costal and subcostal veins light yellow.
11. Shape of discoidal cell in fore wing.
12. Hind wing pterostigma shorter than fore wing.

GENUS *CROCOTHEMIS* BRAUER

The genus *Crocothemis* is raised by Brauer in 1868. It is found throughout continental Africa, Madagaser, S. Europe, Arabia, Mesopotamia, India, S. China, Japan, S. Asia, the sundale Archipelago, New Guinea, Philippines and Australia. Two species have been reported from India. The species of this genus breed in still water but occasionally in the beds of streams during the dry season. They are bright sun loving insects. They are found quite abundant even in small weedy tanks.

The genus shows following characters -

1. These are usually coloured uniform red and with hyaline wings.
2. Head of moderate size; eyes shortly contiguous.
3. Frons with deep sulcus which divides two flattened, slopping, hourseshoe-shaped surfaces; vesicle rounded, low.
4. Prothorax with small posterior lobe; thorax robust; leg rather short, robust, hind femora with numerous closely set small spines of uniform size and a longer one at distal end.

5. Abdomen depressed, moderately broad to broad at base and tapered gradually to the end in male, cylindrical in the female.
6. Wings hyaline or partly coloured at extreme base; reticulation close; long and narrow, pointed at apices; discoidal cell in fore wing narrow, costal side straight, one half the length of distal and basal sides, transversed; discoidal cell of hind wing with base at level of arc, usually entire; sectors of arc shortly fused in fore wing, with a long fusion at origin in the fore; arc situated between the 1st and 2nd antenodal nervures; 7½ to 14½ antenodal nervures, pterostigma and membrane large.

Genotype–*Libellula servilia,* Drury.

Crocothemis Brauer, Verh. Zool. bot. Ges., Wien, Vol. xviii, pp. 367, 736 (1868); Kirby, Trans. Zool, Soc. Lond. Vol. xii, pp 263, 279 (1889); id., Cat. Odon. p. 21 (1890); Forster, Jber. Manmheim, Vols. lxxi, lxxii, pp. 12 (sep.) (1906); Ris, Cat. Coll. Selys, fasc. ix p. 29 (1909); id., ibid. fasc. xiii, pp 532, 533 (1911); Fraser J. Bombay Nat. Hist. Soc. Vol. xxvi, pp. 515-516 (1919).

Beblicia Kirby, Ann. Mag. Nat. Hist., (7) Vol. p. 71 (1900).

CROCOTHEMIS SERVILIA ERYTHREA (BRULLE)

Libellula ferruginea Vander Linden. Mon. Lab. Eur. p. 13 (1825); Fonscolombe, Ann. Soc. Ent. France, Vol. vi, p. 142 (1837); Burmeister, Handb. Ent. Vol. ii, p. 858 (1839); Selys, Mon. Lib. Eur. pp. 27, 42, 207 (1840); Rambur, Ins. Nevrop. p. 79 (1842); Schneider, Stett. Ent. Zeit. Vol. vi, p. iii (1845); id., ibid. Vol. vi, p. 339 (1845): Brittinger, S.B. Akad. Wiss. Wien. vol. iv, p. 332 (1850).

Libellula erythrxa Brulle, Exped. Morec. Vol. iii, (I) p. 102, pl. xxxii, Figure 4 (1832); Hagen, Stett. Ent. Zeit. vol. x p. 69 (1849) (Brulles typen existeren nicht mehr.); Selys. Rev. Odon. pp. 24, 382 (1850), etc.

Libellula coccinea Charpentier, Lib. Eur. p. 70, pl. vii, Figure (1840); Hagen, Syn. Lib. Eur. p. 28 (1840).

Libellula inquinata Rambur, Ins. Nevrop. p. 86 (1842); Selys, Pollan and Van Dam, Madagas. Ins. p. 22 (1869).

Crocothemis inquinata Brauer, Verh. Zool., bot. Ges. Wien., vol. xviii, p. 737 (1868); Kirby, Cat. Odon. p. 22 (1890).

Crocothemis erythraea Brauer, Verh. Zool. bot. Ges. Wien., vol. xviii, p. 737 (1868); Calvert, Proc. Acad. Phil. p. 153 (1898); Morton, Trans. Ent. Soc. Lond. p. 304 (1907); Ris Cat. Coll. Selys, Fascs xiii and xvi, pp. 533, 536, 539, 1165 (1911-1913) (For further and complete list of references consult this last); Fraser, J. Bombay Nat. Hist. Soc. Vol. xxvi, p. 516 (1919); Morton, Ent. Month. Mag. (3) Vol. V. pp. 186, 187 (1919).

Crocothemis servilia servilia var. *erythraea* Fraser, J. Bombay Nat. Hist. Soc. Vol. xxvi, p. 517 (1919).

Orthetrum lorti Kirby Proc. Zool. Soc. Lond. p. 522 (1896).

CROCOTHEMIS SERVILIA ERYTHREA (BRULLE)

MALE (Figures 12,13)

Body 35.00 mm long excluding anal appendages; head 3.00 mm, thorax 11.00 mm long, fore wing 25.00 mm long, hind wing 24.00 mm long; abdomen 21.00 mm long, reddish yellow, anal appendages 1.30 mm long with yellowish black.

HEAD

3.00 mm long, 5.00 mm broad, roughly circular; occiput yellowish; compound eyes blackish brown, occular space 2.5 mm, three ocelli in triangle, black; ocellar space 0.24 mm; interocellar space 0.90 mm; frons reddish with deep sulcus, postclypeus yellowish, anteclypeus yellowish, labrum brownish, mandibles black, mandible bases brownish, labium yellowish.

Antenna

1.56 mm long, 0.10 mm broad (width of scape 0.10 mm), black, 6 segmented; scape 0.06 mm long, 0.10 mm broad; pedicel 0.24 mm long, 0.08 mm broad. Flagellum: 4 segmented, 1.24 mm long, 0.04 mm broad; 1st segment 0.30 mm long, 0.04 mm broad; 2nd segment 0.34 mm long, 0.034 mm broad; 3rd segment 0.28 mm long, 0.023 mm broad; 4th segment 0.34 mm long, 0.014 mm broad.

Flagellar Formula

L/W; ½ = 7.5/10; $^{2/2}$ = 10/10; $^{3/2}$ = 12.17/10; $^{4/2}$ = 24.28/10; A = 1.074.

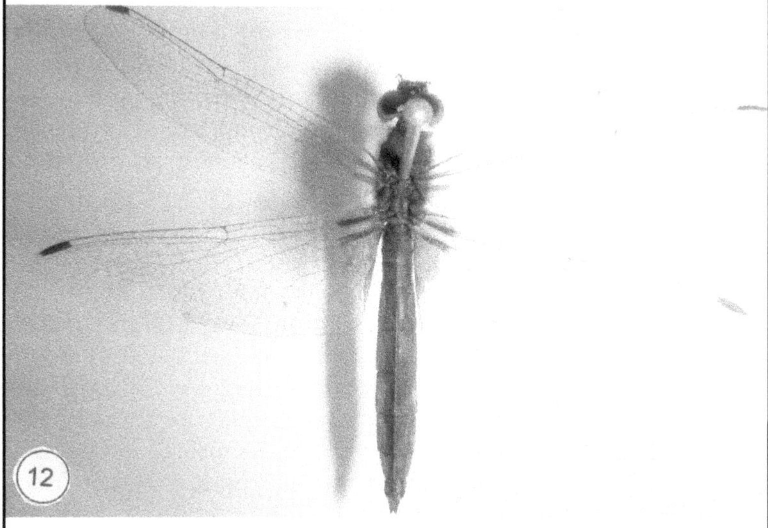

Figure 12: *Crocothemis servilia erythrea*, Male

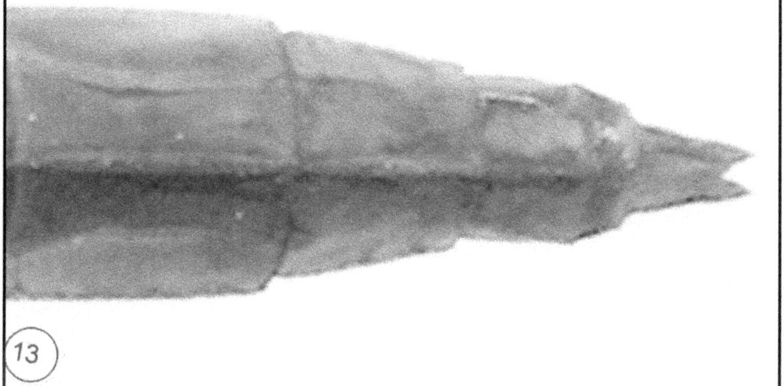

Figure 13: *Crocothemis servilia erythrea:*
Anal Appendages; Male

THORAX

11.00 mm long, 4.00 mm broad, yellowish brown with dense hairs; prothorax 6.00 mm long, 4.00 mm broad; yellowish brown with dense hairs with 3 lobes; anterior lobe 0.7 mm long, blackish; middle lobe 5.00 mm long, 4.00 mm broad, yellowish brown with dense hairs; posterior lobe 0.3 mm long, 4.00 mm broad, brownish; synthorax 5.00 mm long, 4.00 mm broad, yellowish brown on dorsolaterally.

WINGS

Wings hyaline, wing apices black, pointed, reticulation close, wing venation black. Fore wing: 25.00 mm long, 7.00 mm broad; 53.00 mm wing span, pterostigma 1.90 mm long, 0.70 mm broad, brownish; antenodal nervures 13, post nodal nervures 11; wing bases with orange patch. Hind wing: 24.00 mm long, 9.00 mm broad; 51.00 mm wing span, pterostigma 1.86 mm long, 0.70 mm broad, brownish, antenodal nervures 10, postnodal nervures 11, wing bases with large orange patch.

LEG

Hind leg: 12.00 mm long, 0.80 mm broad (width of coxa 0.80 mm); coxa 0.60 mm long, 0.80 mm broad, yellow with yellowish hairs on outer side; trochanter 2 segmented; 1st segment 0.50 mm long, 0.40 mm broad; yellowish; 2nd segment 0.90 mm long, 0.40 mm broad; 0.40 mm part of trochanter overlaps on femora, yellowish; femora 3.70 mm long, 0.50 mm broad, black with thin, yellow hairs on inner side; tibia 4.20 mm long, 0.24 mm broad, yellow with thin, black, pointed spines on inner side, spine 0.32 mm long; tarsus 3 segmented, black with spines; 1st segment 0.60 mm long, 0.14 mm broad; 2nd segment 0.50 mm long, 0.12 mm broad; 3rd segment 0.40 mm long, 0.14 mm broad; claws 0.60 mm long, 0.12 mm broad, reddish.

ABDOMEN

21.00 mm long, 2.40 mm broad, yellowish orange red segment 1st, 2nd, reddish, segment 3rd reddish with black transverse ring, segment 4, 5, 6 and 8 brownish, segment 9th brownish with blackish tinge, segment 10th anterior 2/3 part black and posterior 1/3 brown. Segment 8th and 9th without black marking on mid dorsal carina.

Anal Appendages (Figure 13)

Yellow.

COLOUR

Blackish brown: Compound eyes.

Black: Ocelli, mandibles, femora, tarsus

Reddish: Frons.

Brownish: Labrum

Yellowish: Labium, occiput.

Yellowish brown: Thorax.

Yellow: Coxa, trochanter, tibia.

PREY RECORD: Pyralid moth, mosquitoes.

HOLOTYPE: Male, India, Maharashtra, Coll. 2, 26-IX-2004, Munawale, Satara district, M.S. Shinde, K.P., antenna, leg on slide labelled as above, other parts with pined form, labelled as above.

PARATYPE: Male 1, coll. 23-I-2005, same data as above.

DISTRIBUTIONAL RECORD/OBSERVATIONS

Male 70, female 7. Patan ♂7, 10-X-2004; Yerad ♂10, 19-XII-2004; Kadoli ♂10, ♀3, 3-IV-2005; Tapola ♂2♀2, 15-V-2005; Rohine ♂15♀1, 22-V-2005; Morgiri ♂5, 12-II-2006; Ghatmatha ♂3♀1, 30-IV-2006.

CROCOTHEMIS SERVILIA SERVILIA (DRURY)

MALE (Figures 14,15)

Body 44.00 mm in length excluding anal appendages, head 4.00 mm long, thorax 13.00 mm long, fore wing 35.00 mm long, hind wing 33.00 mm long, abdomen 27.00 mm long, blood red with black patch on dorsal side; anal appendages 1.40 mm long, yellow with black tip.

HEAD

4.00 mm long, 6.50 mm broad, roughly rounded; occiput brown, compound eyes blood red or blackish, ocellar space 3.25 mm; three ocelli in triangle, black with basally yellow ring, ocellar space 0.22 mm, interocellar space 0.90 mm; frons dark black with deep sulcus; postclypeus reddish with two black spots on front side; anteclypeus

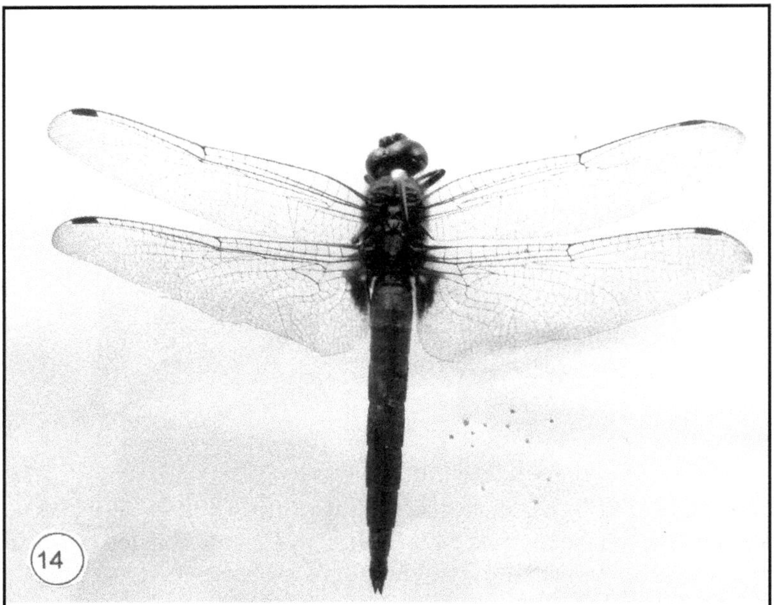

Figure 14: ***Crocothermis servilia servilia*; Male**

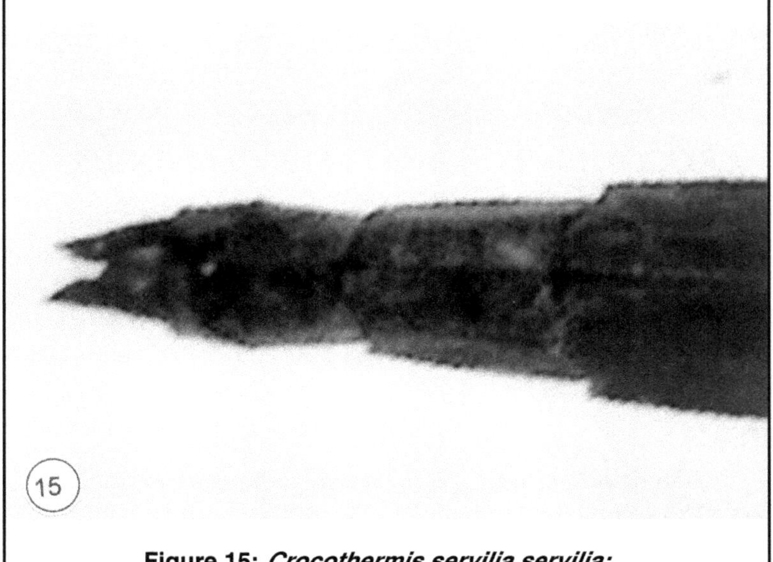

Figure 15: ***Crocothermis servilia servilia:***
Anal Appendages; Male

reddish yellow; labrum black, mandible brown, mandible bases reddish, labium dark brown.

Antenna

1.54 mm long, 0.16 mm broad (width of scape 0.16 mm); 6 segmented, black; scape 0.06 mm long, 0.16 mm broad; pedicel 0.30 mm long, 0.14 mm broad. Flagellum: 4 segmented, 1.18 mm long, 0.06 mm broad; 1st segment 0.30 mm long, 0.06 mm broad; 2nd segment 0.22 mm long, 0.042 mm broad; 3rd segment 0.24 mm long, 0.017 mm broad; 4th segment 0.42 mm long, 0.010 mm broad.

Flagellar Formula

L/W; ½ = 5/5.23; $^{2/2}$ = 5.25/5.25; $^{3/2}$ = 14.11/5.23; $^{4/2}$ = 42/5.23; A = 2.53.

THORAX

13.00 mm long, 6.00 mm broad, bluish with dense hairs; prothorax 7.00 mm long, 6.00 mm broad, bluish with dense hairs and three lobed; anterior lobe 0.9 mm long, black with dense white hairs transversely, middle lobe 5.8 mm long, 6.00 mm broad, bluish with dense hairs and middorsally black stripe; posterior lobe 0.3 mm long, 6.00 mm broad, bluish with dense hairs; synthorax 6.00 mm long, 6.00 mm broad, robust dorsally and bluish dorsolaterally.

WINGS (Figure 14)

Wing hyaline, wing apices brown, yellowish tinge on both fore wing and hind wing apically, reticulation close, wing venation black; wing bases marked with rich ambur yellow. Fore wing: 35.00 mm long, 11.00 mm broad, 73.00 mm wing span; pterostigma 2.80 mm long, 0.60 mm broad, blackish brown with black border; antenodal neruvres 13, post nodal nervures 9. Hind wing: 33.00 mm long, 8.00 mm broad, 69.00 mm wing span; pterostigma 2.80 mm long, 0.70 mm broad, blackish brown with dark black border; antenodal nervures 11, postnodal nervures 10, mahogany.

LEG

Hind leg 18.90 mm long, 1.20 mm broad (width of coxa 1.20 mm); coxa 2.40 mm long, 1.20 mm broad, reddish brown with dense hairs; trochanter 2 segmented 2.60 mm long, 0.62 mm broad, reddish; 1st segment 0.80 mm long, 0.50 mm broad, reddish; 2nd segment 1.80 mm long, 0.62 mm broad, reddish; 0.55 mm part of trochanter overlaps on femora; femora 4.80 mm long, 0.72 mm broad, black with 22 blunt spines and many yellowish long, thin spines; tibia–5.00 mm long, 0.32 mm broad; 7 long, pointed, thick spines, spine length 0.60 mm and small pointed spines on outer side; tarsus 3 segmented, 3.30 mm long, 0.28 mm broad, black; 1st segment 0.90 mm long, 0.24 mm broad, black with 5 spines on inner side; 2nd segment 1.10 mm long, 0.28 mm broad, black with 10 spines on inner side; 3rd segment 1.30 mm long, 0.22 mm broad, black with 8 spines on inner side; claws 0.80 mm long, 0.20 mm broad with 4 spines.

ABDOMEN (Figure 15)

27.00 mm long, 4.00 mm broad, yellowish brown. 1st segment yellowish brown, 2nd and 3rd blood red; 3, 4 and 5 segment blood red with black patches on dorsal side; segment 6, 7, 8 and 9 red with black spots, segment 10 yellow. Anal appendages (Figure 15): Red blood colour, superior anal appendages 1.40 mm long, 0.28 mm broad, blood red with dense hairs and black at tip; inferior anal appendages 0.80 mm long, 0.36 mm broad, yellow with black tip.

COLOUR

Red: Abdomen.

Reddish: Trochanter.

Blood Red: Anal appendages.

Bluish: Thorax.

Brown: Labrum, ocelli, tibia, tarsus

Black: Frons

PREY RECORD: Mosquitoes *Aedes* sp., *Culex* sp., *Anopheles* sp., Moths *Chilo* spp.

HOLOTYPE: Male, India, Maharashtra, Coll.2, 19-XII-2004; Kadoli, Satara district, M.S., Shinde, K.P., antenna, leg on slide labelled as above, other parts with pined form, labelled as above.

PARATYPE: Male 1, Coll. 10-X-2004; same data as above.

DISTRIBUTIONAL RECORD/OBSERVATIONS

Male, 40, female 2. Kamargaon ♂7 ♀1, 3-X-2004; Bamnoli ♂5, 5-XII-2004; Navaja ♂8, 6-III-2005; Morgiri ♂7, 3-VII-2005; Patan ♂10 ♀1, 4-XI-2005; Kargaon ♂3, 30-IV-2006.

GENUS *TRITHEMIS* BRAUER

The genus *Trithemis* is raised by Brauer in 1868. This genus is distributed in Ethopian and Oriental region, extending to Formosa, Borneo and Philippines. This is large genus however, only four species have been reported from India and all commonly distributed except *T. kirbyi kirbyi,* which is confined to the West Coast of India. One species, *T. pallidinervis,* is decidedly aberant differing not only in some important morphological details but also strongly in its habits; it may possibly require to be placed in a genus of its own. All individuals of this genus breed in still waters or sluggish streams and the larvae found hiding up in masses of water weed.

The genus is characterised by having following features:

1. Dragonflies of medium size, variable in colour and shape.
2. Head small or average size.
3. Eyes moderately contiguous.
4. Frons variable, with or without a distinct crest, vesicle broad, depressed.
5. Prothorax with a small posterior lobe, not fringed with hairs; thorax rather narrow;
6. Legs variable, moderately long and robust or very long and slim; hind femora with a row of very closely-set small spines and a single, much longer one at distant end;
7. Abdomen variable in the species;
8. Wings long and relatively broad, reticulation usually close, discoidal cell of fore wing narrow, costal side about half the length of proximal transversed. Hind wing with base at level of arc, entire subtrigone of fore wing 3 celled; sectors of arc with a long fusion at origin. 8½ to 15½ antenodal nervures in fore wing.
9. Pterostigma short, membrane rather long.

Trithemis Brauer, verh, Zool. bot, Ges. wien, vol., xviii, p. 176 (1868); Kirby, Trans. Zool. Soc. Lond, vol. xii, pp. 264, 277 (1889); Karsch, Berlin Ent, Zeit. vol., xxxiii, p. 357 (1890); Kirby, Cat. Odon. p. 18 (1890): Ris Ent. News, vol. xiv. p. 218 (1903): Needham, Proc. U.S. Nat. Mus. vol. xxvi, pl. 1 Figure 1 (1903); Forster, Jber. Mannheim, vols. lxxi, lxxii, p. 12 (Sep.) (1906): Ris. Cat. Coll. Selys, Fascs. ix and xiv, pp. 33 757-762 (1909-1912); Fraser J. Bombay Nat. Hist. Soc. vol. xxvi, pp. 919, 920 (1920) Stoechia Kirby (pars), Ann. Mag. Nat. Hist. (7) Vol. ii, p. 235 (1898).

TRITHEMIS MAHARASHTRI SP.NOV.

MALE (Figures 16, 17)

34.00 mm body length excluding anal appendages; head 3.00 mm long, thorax 8.00 mm long; fore wing 30.00 mm long, hind wing 29.00 mm long; abodmen 23.00 mm long, black; anal appendages 1.5 mm long, black with hairs.

HEAD

3.00 mm long, 5.00 mm broad, roughly rounded, occiput black with white hairs, compound eyes broadly contiguous with blackish brown, occular space 2.5 mm; three ocelli in triangle, ocellar space 0.12 mm; interocellar space 0.96 mm; frons dark black with dense black hairs and two pink spots; postclypeus brown; anteclypeus brown, labrum black, mandible black, bases of mandible brown, labium brown with black patch.

Antenna

1.23 mm long, 0.12 mm broad (width of scape 0.12 mm), black; scape 0.05 mm long, 0.12 mm broad; pedicel 0.22 mm long, 0.10 mm broad; Flagellum: 5 segmented, 0.93 mm long, 0.4 mm broad; 1st segment 0.14 mm long, 0.04 mm broad; 2nd segment 0.12mm long, 0.031 mm broad; 3rd segment 0.24 mm long, 0.017 mm broad; 4th segment 0.22 mm long, 0.07 mm broad; 5th segment 0.24 mm long, 0.009 mm broad.

Flagellar Formula

L/W; ½ = 3.5/3.87; $^{2/2}$ = 3.87/3.87; $^{3/2}$ = 14.11/3.87; $^{4/2}$ = 3.14/ 3.87; $^{5/2}$ = 26.66/3.87; A = 2.64.

THORAX

8.00 mm long, 4.00 mm broad, brown with dense long hairs on entire thorax; prothorax 4.80 mm long, 4.00 mm broad, brown with dense black, long hairs, 3 lobed; anterior lobe 0.3 mm long, black with white hairs; mid lobe 4.50 mm long, 4.00 mm broad, brown with black, dense, long hairs on entire lobe and mid dorsally small

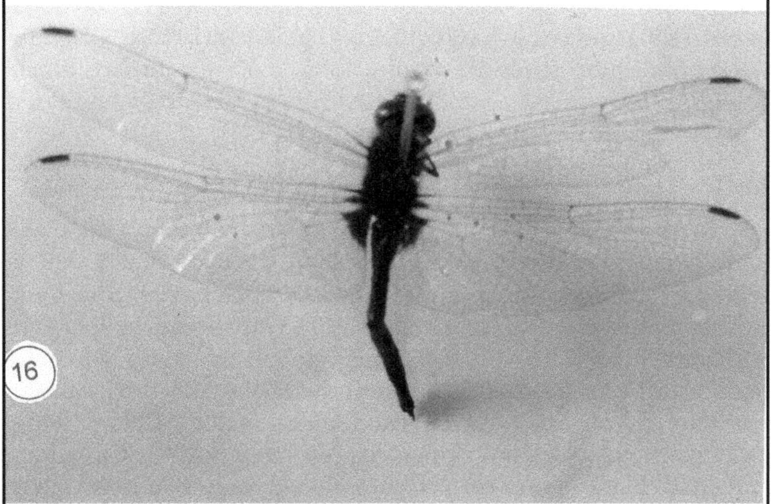

Figure 16: ***Trithemis maharashtri*** **sp.nov.; Male**

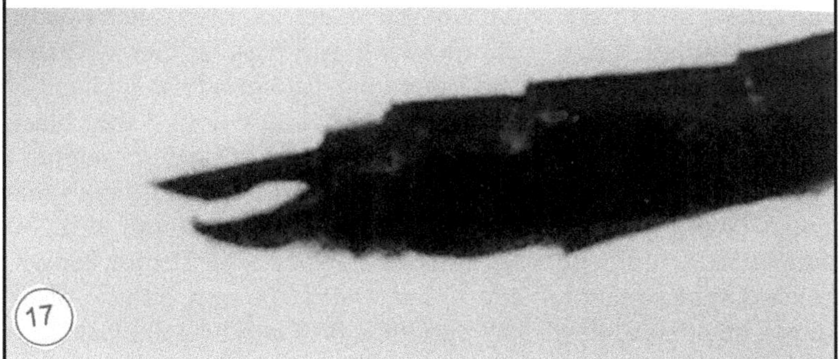

Figure 17: ***Trithemis maharashtri:*** **Anal Appendages; Male**

narrow yellowish plate; posterior lobe 0.2 mm long, 4.00 mm broad, plate like structure brown and hairy; synthorax robust, blackish brown, hairy with one yellow spot.

WINGS

Wings hyaline, wing apices black, pointed; close reticulation, black venation, pterostigma equal in length in both wings. Fore wing:

30.00 mm long, 7.00 mm broad, 63.00 mm wing span; pterostigma 2.46 mm long, 0.6 mm broad, black; antenodal nervures 11, postnodal nervures 9. Hind wing: 58.00 mm long, 10.00 mm broad; 62.00 mm wing span; pterostigma 2.44 mm long, 0.60 mm broad, black; antenodal nervures 9, postnodal nervures 10; wing bases rounded with mahogany or dark brown mark.

LEG

14.38 mm long, 0.80 mm broad (width of coxa 0.80 mm), black with hairs and spines; coxa 1.50 mm long, 0.80 mm broad, yellow with 18 long hairs inner side; hairs long, black, 0.58 mm long; trochanter 2 segmented, 1.60 mm long, 0.38 mm broad, yellow with few hairs outer side, hairs 0.40 mm long and few inner side hairs black, basal hairs length 0.30 mm and apex hairs 0.08 mm long; 0.40 mm part of trochanter overlaps on femora; femora 4.08 mm long, 0.42 mm broad, black with inner side few hairs, hairs 0.50 mm long and small black spines on surface in which only two long one in length 0.10 mm and another 0.52 mm on outer side, only 3 small black pointed spines; spines 0.08 mm long, tibia 4.60 mm long, 0.22 mm broad, black with 11 pairs of thin, black, pointed downwardly directed spines, spines 0.22 mm long and basal spines 0.52 mm long; tarsus 3 segmented, 2.12 mm long, 0.16 mm broad, black; 1st segment 0.62 mm long, 0.16 mm broad, black with 2 thin black pointed spines on outer side and 6 spines inner side; 2nd segment 0.60 mm long, 0.12 mm broad, with 6 thin spines on outer side, spine length 0.06 mm, 5 thick, pointed black spines on outer side; 3rd segment 0.90 mm long, 0.08 mm broad, black with 11 thin, brown, pointed spines on outer side, spine length 0.06 mm, 5 thick, black spines inner side; claws 0.48 mm long, 0.12 mm broad, black with only two spines.

ABDOMEN

23.00 mm long, 2.2 mm broad, black with broad anteriorly and narrowly tapering posteriorly; 1st segment broad and black; 2nd segment black with brown hairs, 3, 4 segments black, 5, 6 and 7 segments black with 2 brown spots on dorsal side for each segment; 9 and 10 black with yellow ring on basal side and with yellow hairs. Anal appendages (Figure 17): Black, superior 1.50 mm long, 0.20 mm broad, with dense hairs; inferior anal appendages 1.06 mm long, 0.46 mm broad, triangular black with few hairs.

COLOUR

Black: Abdomen, anal appendages, tarsus, occiput, frons, mandible, labrum.

Brown: Postclypeus, anteclypeus, labium

Yellow: Coxa, trochanter.

PREY RECORD: Mosquitoes *Culex* sp.

HOLOTYPE: Male, India, Maharashtra, Coll. 2, 14-XI-2004; Khirkhindi, Satara district, M.S., Shinde, K.P., antenna, leg on slide, labelled as above.

PARATYPE: Male 1, Coll. 10-X-2004; same data as above.

DISTRIBUTIONAL RECORD/OBSERVATIONS

Male 14, female 1. Munawale ♂2, 3-X-2004; Kadoli ♂1, 26-XII-2004; Dara ♂1 ♀1, 13-II-2005; Morgiri ♂2 10-IV-2005; Tapola ♂3, 8-V-2005; Kusawade ♂3, 11-XI-2005; Kusapur ♂2, 22-I-2006.

DISCUSSION

The species *Trithemis maharashtri* sp.nov. known runs close to *Trithemis festiva* (Rambur) by following characters -

1. Labium brown.
2) Labrum black.
3. Legs black.

However, it differs from above species by having following characters:

1. Frons dark black.
2. Occiput black.
3. Prothorax not dark blue but brown.
4. Wing bases.
5. Fore wing antenodal nervures 11; postnodal nervures 9.
6. Hind wing antenodal nervures 9; postnodal nervures 10.
7. Anal appendages black but lanciolate.
8. Flagellar formula: L/W; ½ = 3.5/3.87; $^{2/2}$ = 3.87/3.87; $^{3/2}$ = 14.11/3.87; $^{4/2}$ = 3.14/3.87; $^{5/2}$ = 26.66/3.87; A = 2.64.
9. Nervures in between anal and cubital region.

TRITHEMIS FESTIVA (RAMBUR)

MALE (Figures 18, 19)

49.00 mm body length excluding anal appendages, head 4.00 mm long, thorax 14.00 mm long, fore wing 29.00 mm long, hind wing 30.00 mm long; abdomen 31.00 mm long, blackish brown; superior anal appendages 1.12 mm long, black with dense hairs.

HEAD

4.00 mm long, 7.00 mm broad, roughly rounded, occiput dark brown, compound eyes broadly contiguous with blackish brown colour, occular space 3.5 mm; three ocelli in triangle, brown anterior ocellar space 0.24 mm, posterior ocellar space 0.42 mm, interocellar space 0.86 mm; frons robust black; postclypeus brown; anteclypeus brown; labrum black with base brown; mandible black, mandible bases brown; labium blackish brown.

Antenna

1.64 mm long, 0.18 mm broad (width of scape 0.18 mm), black with basal yellow rings; scape 0.04 mm long, 0.18 mm broad; pedicel 0.24 mm long, 0.16 mm broad; Flagellum: 5 segmented, 1.36 mm long, 0.06 mm broad; 1st segment 0.34 mm long, 0.06 mm broad; 2nd segment 0.18 mm long, 0.04 mm broad; 3rd segment 0.28 mm long, 0.029 mm broad; 4th segment 0.36 mm long, 0.014 mm broad; 5th segment 0.20 mm long, 0.008 mm broad.

Flagellar Formula

L/W; ½ = 5.66/4.5; $^{2/2}$ = 4.5/4.5; $^{3/2}$ = 9.65/4.5; $^{4/2}$ = 25.71/4.5; $^{5/2}$ = 25/4.5; A = 3.13.

THORAX

14.00 mm long, 6.00 mm broad, robust, yellowish with dense hairs; prothorax 8.00 mm long, 6.00 mm broad, dark blue with dense hairs and 3 lobed; anterior lobe 0.7 mm broad, yellow with black margin and dense yellow hairs; mid lobe 7.00 mm long, 4.00 mm broad, blackish with dense hairs and on dorsal blackish; posterior lobe 0.3 mm long, 6.00 mm broad with black band; synthorax 6.00 mm long, 6.00 mm broad, dorsally robust, laterally one black and one yellow band.

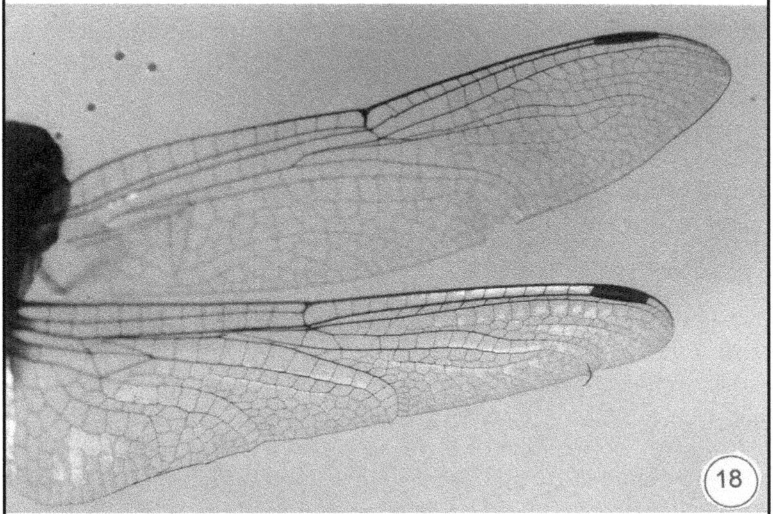

Figure 18: ***Trithemis festiva*; Male**

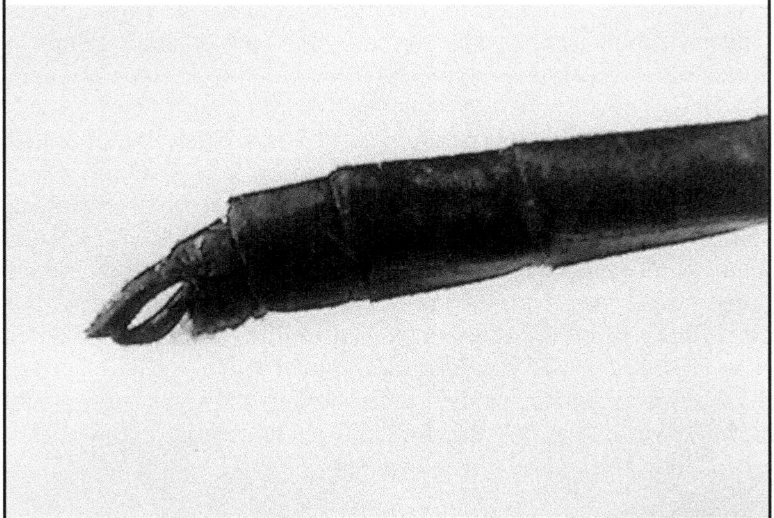

Figure 19: ***Trithemis festiva:*** **Anal Appendages; Male**

WINGS

Wings hyaline, wing apices brown and pointed; close reticulation, black venation, brown costal border; round bases; fore wing 29.00 mm long, 8.00 mm broad, 62.00 mm wing span, pterostigma 2.70 mm long, 0.74 mm broad, black; antenodal nervures 15, postnodal nervures 11; Hind wing: 30.00 mm long, 12.00 mm broad; 64.00 mm wing span; pterostigma 2.66 mm long, 0.60 mm broad, black, antenodal nervures 11, postnodal nervures 14, hind wings with dark opaque brown mark at base.

LEG

Hind leg 20.26 mm long, 1.10 mm broad (width of coxa 1.10 mm); black with spines and hairs; coxa 2.20 mm long, 1.10 mm broad, yellowish red with few brown hairs outer side, hair length 0.38 mm inner side bunch of yellow hairs, hair length 0.52 mm; trochanter 2 segmented, 2.44 mm long, 0.58 mm broad, black few hairs and spines; 1st segment 0.90 mm long, 0.52 mm broad, black with red patch and 3 small spines and few hairs, spine 0.04 mm long, hairs 0.24 mm long; 2nd segment 1.54 mm long, 0.58 mm broad; black with red patch, no hairs and spines, 0.96 mm part of trochanter overlaps on femora; femora 5.88 mm long, 0.60 mm broad, black with red small patches, also on both side row of small spines in which outer side spines, spines of inner side black, thick pointed, last 3 long, spine length 0.18 mm; tibia 5.60 mm long, 0.42 mm broad, black with red and yellow patch with 11 pairs of black, thick, pointed spines on inner side, spines on basal region long, 0.42 mm long; tarsus black, 3 segmented, 3.28 mm long, 0.24 mm broad with black spines; 1st segment 0.86 mm long, 0.24 mm broad, black with 4 black, thick, blunt spines inner side and 3 pointed, thin, yellow spines outer side; 2nd segment 0.96 mm long and 0.24 mm broad with 6 black, thick, blunt spines inner side and 5 thin, yellow spines outer side; 3rd segment 1.46 mm long, 0.26 mm broad, black with 7 black thick blunt spines inner side, 5 yellow thin small spines outer side; claws 0.86 mm long, 0.26 mm broad, black with red tip; claws black with 2 long spines and 2 small spines.

ABDOMEN

31.00 mm long, 3.00 mm broad; black, 1st segment black with yellow spot on dorsal side; 2nd segment yellowish, 3rd segment blackish brown with three black rings; segment 4, 5, 6 blackish brown, segment 8, 9, 10 blackish brown with white hairs. Anal appendages (Figure 19): Black, like libelluline shape, superior anal appendages 1.12 mm long, 0.32 mm broad, black with dense hairs, lanciolate; inferior anal appendages 1.00 mm long, 0.30 mm broad, triangular.

COLOUR

Blackish brown: Abdomen, compound eyes

Black: Frons, labrum mandible legs; labium, thorax.

Brown: Occiput, anteclypeus, postclypeus.

Dark blue: Prothorax.

PREY RECORD: Moths, *Chilo* spp.

HOLOTYPE: Male, India, Maharashtra, Coll. 2, 7-XI-2004; Korgaon, Satara district, M.S., Shinde K.P., antenna, leg on slide, labelled as above, other parts with pined form, labelled as above.

PARATYPE: Male 1, Coll. 19-XII-2004, same data as above.

DISTRIBUTIONAL RECORD/OBSERVATIONS

Male 17, female 2. Munawale ♂1,♀1‹ 21-XI-2004; Kamargaon ♂1, 6-II-2005; Nisare ♂2, 3-IV-2005; Ghatmatha ♂1♀1, 8-V-2005; Yerad ♂3, 4-IX-2005; Kadoli ♂5, 6-X-2005; Morgiri ♂2, 5-II-2006; Khirkhindi ♂1, 19-III-2006; Patan ♂1, 7-V-2006.

TRITHEMIS HIVEI SP.NOV.

MALE (Figures 20, 21)

43.00 mm in body length excluding anal appendages, head 5 mm long, thorax 12.00 mm long, fore wing 38 mm long, hind wing 36.00 mm long; abdomen 26.00 mm long, yellow, anal appendages 1.70 mm long, yellow with black tip.

HEAD

5.00 mm long, 7.00 mm broad, roughly triangular; occiput brown, compound eyes red on dorsal side with blackish patches on lateral side but not brownish and front pink on ventrolateral side but not bluish grey ventrally. Occular space 3.5 mm; three ocelli in triangle, black; ocellar space 0.24 mm, interocellar space 1.10 mm; frons yellow, postclypeus faint yellow; anteclypeus faint yellow

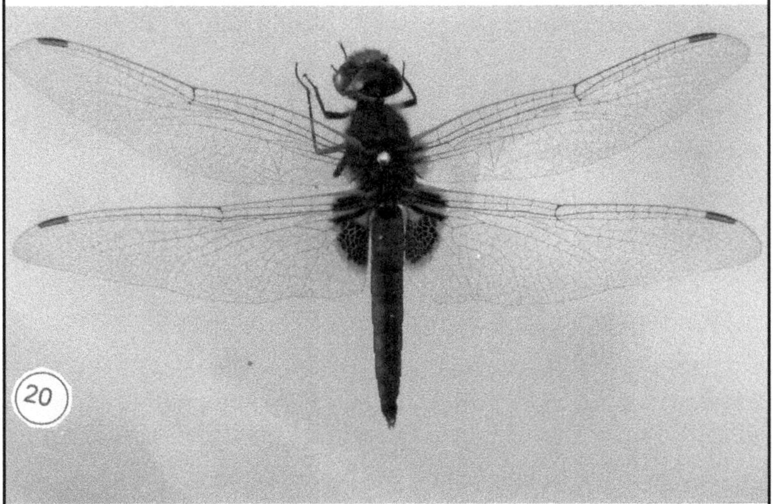

Figure 20: *Trithemis hivei* sp.nov.; Male

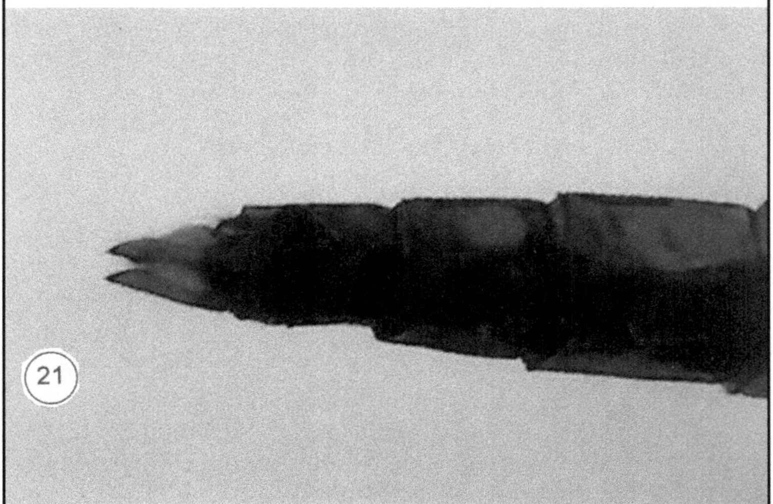

Figure 21: *Trithemis hivei:* Anal Appendages; Male

brownish; labrum faint red; mandible reddish brown; bases of mandible reddish yellow, labium reddish with basal border black with white hairs.

Antenna

2.68 mm long, 0.24 mm broad (width of scape 0.24 mm), black, 7 segmented; scape 0.12 mm long, 0.24 mm broad; pedicel 0.40 mm long, 0.20 mm broad; Flagellum: 5 segmented, 2.16 mm long, 0.06 mm broad, black with yellow rings; 1st segment 0.60 mm long, 0.06 mm broad; 2nd segment 0.56 mm long, 0.04 mm broad; 3rd segment 0.28 mm long, 0.034 mm broad; 4th segment 0.32 mm long, 0.022 mm broad; 5th segment 0.40 mm long, 0.009 mm broad.

Flagellar Formula

L/W; ½ = 10/14; $^{2/2}$ = 14/14; $^{3/2}$ = 8.23/14; $^{4/2}$ = 14.54/14; $^{5/2}$ = 44/14; A = 1.29.

THORAX

12.00 mm long, 6.00 mm broad, yellowish with yellow dense hairs on dorsal and lateral sides; prothorax 5.00 mm long, 6.00 mm broad, dull brown red with dense yellow hairs on dorsal, lateral and ventral surface; prothorax 3 lobed, anterior lobe 0.4 mm long, black but not yellow with white hairs; mid lobe 4.3 mm long, 6.00 mm broad, yellowish with yellow hairs, dorsal side with blackish tinge and on mid dorsal side red line; posterior lobe 0.3 mm long, 6.00 mm broad, dorsal side with dark yellowish line, ventral side yellowish with black tinge; synthorax 7.00 mm long, 6.00 mm broad, yellowish with one reddish spot and two small blackish stripes on lateral side but not three, dorsally robust.

WINGS

Wings hyaline, wing apices brown and pointed; reticulation close and yellowish but not reddish, wing venation yellowish and bright amber yellow basal marking, Fore wing: 38.00 mm long, 8.00 mm broad, 79.00 mm wing span, basal wing venation yellow with basal side yellow spot; pterostigma 3.20 mm long, 0.70 mm broad, yellow with faint black border; antenodal nervures 8½, postnodal nervures 8; Hind wing: 36.00 mm long, 12.00 mm broad, 75.00 mm wing span; basal wing venation yellow with brownish yellow patches on the bases except costa. Anal margin with mahogany dark black patch with yellow nervure. The marking extends upto antenodal nervures, same patch bordered by yellow colour patch beehive like in appearance; pterostigma 3.50 mm long, 0.68 mm broad with dark black border; antenodal nervures 6½, post nodal nervure 8.

LEG

Hind leg 20.86 mm long, 1.40 mm broad (width of coxa 1.40 mm), black; coxa 1.10 mm long, 1.40 mm broad, yellowish, red with yellow hairs, hairs 0.42 mm long; trochanter 2 segmented, 2.00 mm long, 0.60 mm broad; 1st segment 0.60 mm long 0.42 mm broad and yellow, anterior side brown, few hairs on 1st segment; 2nd segment 1.40 mm long, 0.60 mm broad, brown with few hairs on outer side; 0.60 mm part of trochanter overlaps on femora; femora 6.24 mm long, 0.70 mm broad, reddish black with very small spines on outer side and on inner side few hairs and few small spines but only one large spine at basal region, measuring 0.38 mm in length; tibia: 7.60 mm long, 0.34 mm broad, reddishblack, with black pointed 11 spines on inner side, spine length 0.42 mm, on outer side very small spines; tarsus 3 segmented, 3.20 mm long, 0.30 mm broad, black pointed, with thick spines; 1st segment 1.00 mm long, 0.30 mm broad, black with 6 long spines on inner side, spines 0.28 mm long and outer side very thin brown with pointed spines; 2nd segment 0.90 mm long, black, with black pointed 6 spines on inner side, few small pointed brown spines on outer side; 3rd segment 1.30 mm long 0.26 mm broad, black with 7 spines inner side, spines black, pointed, 0.22 mm long, on outer side few brown pointed spines; claws 0.72 mm long, 0.22 mm broad with two long and two short pointed spines.

ABDOMEN

26.00 mm long, 3.00 mm broad; yellow with black longitudinal black marking at mid dorsally, abdomen with reddish tinge and dark black spots on dorsal side, 1st segment yellowish with dark black patch on dorsal side, 2nd and 3rd segments large with yellow and with transverse red rings, 4th segment yellowishreddish and with one black triangular mark; 5th, 6th, 7th, 8th and 9th segment yellowish with black patch on dorsal side; 10th segment smallest and yellowishred and with black spot on dorsal side. Anal appendages (Figure 21) yellow, tip black, superior anal appendages 1.70 mm long, 0.44 mm broad with dark yellow and few hairs at anterior side, hairs sparely arranged; inferior anal appendages 1.10 mm long, 0.60 mm broad with yellow and with basal black spot.

COLOUR

Brown: Occiput

Yellow: Abdomen, anal appendages, frons

Reddish: Labrum

Yellowish: Thorax

Black: Prothorax

Reddish black: Femora, tibia.

PREY RECORD: Moths, jassids

HOLOTYPE: Male, India, Maharashtra, Coll. 2, 10-X-2004; Patan, Satara district, M.S. Shinde, K.P., antenna, leg on slide labelled as above, other parts with pinned form, labelled as above.

PARATYPE: Male 1, Coll. 13-VI-2005; same data as above.

DISTRIBUTIONAL RECORD/OBSERVATIONS

Morgiri ♂2, 7-XI-2004; Ghatmatha ♂1, 19-XII-2004; Kamargaon ♂2♀1, 9-X-2005; Sodnari ♂3, 4-XII-2005; Nisare ♂1, 25-XII-2005; Munawale ♂2, 1-I-2006; Kusawade ♂2, 7-V-2006; Patan ♂1, 4-VI-2006.

DISCUSSION

This species runs close to *Trithemis pallidinervis* (Kirby) by following characters:

1. Legs longer
2. Eyes reddish brown
3. Thorax coated with grayish hairs

However, it differs from the above species by having following characters:

1. Labium reddish
2. Labrum not black but reddish
3. Reddishbrown eyes with black spots.
4. Flagellar formula: L/W; ½ = 10/14; $^{2/2}$ = 14/14; $^{3/2}$ = 8.23/ 14; $^{4/2}$ = 14.54/14; $^{5/2}$ = 44/14; A = 1.29.

5. Wing hyaline with yellowish reticulation.
6. Pterostigma blackish brown
7. Fore wing–antenodal nervures 8½, post nodal nervures 8.
8. Hind wing–antenodal nervures 6½, post nodal nervures 8.
9. Superior anal appendages not very long lanceolate.

TRITHEMIS PALLIDINERVIS (KIRBY)

MALE (Figure 22, 23)

41.00 mm in body length excluding anal appendages, head 4.00 mm long, thorax 13.00 mm long, fore wing 31.00 mm long, hind wing 29.00 mm long; abdomen 24.00 mm long, reddish yellow with black patches; superior anal appendages 1.70 mm long.

HEAD

4.00 mm long, 6.00 mm broad, roughly circular; occiput olivaceous; compound eyes reddish brown, occular space 3.00 mm; three ocelli in triangle, black; ocellar space 1.16 mm; frons reddish brown; postclypeus pale brown, anteclypeus brown; labrum black; mandible black, mandible bases yellowish; labium yellow.

Antenna

1.64 mm long, 0.14 mm broad, (width of scape 0.14 mm), black; scape 0.08 mm long, 0.14 mm broad; pedicel 0.20 mm long, 0.12 mm broad; Flagellum: 5 segmented, 1.64 mm long, 0.041 mm broad; 1st segment 0.40 mm long, 0.041 mm broad; 2nd segment 0.22 mm long, 0.032 mm broad; 3rd segment 0.26 mm long, 0.017 mm broad; 4th segment 0.12 mm long, 0.001 mm broad; 5th segment 0.36 mm long, 0.007 mm broad.

Flagellar Formula

L/W; ½ = 9.75/6.87; $^{2/2}$ = 6.87/6.87; $^{3/2}$ = 15.29/6.87; $^{4/2}$ = 12/6.87; $^{5/2}$ = 51.42/6.87; A = 2.77.

THORAX

13.00 mm long, 5.50 mm broad, olivaceous-brown on dorsum, brighter olivaceous on lower part, dorsum thickly coated with greyish hairs; a dark brown triangle on mid-dorsum, three black stripes on dorsum; prothorax 6.00 mm long, 5.50 mm broad; prothorax

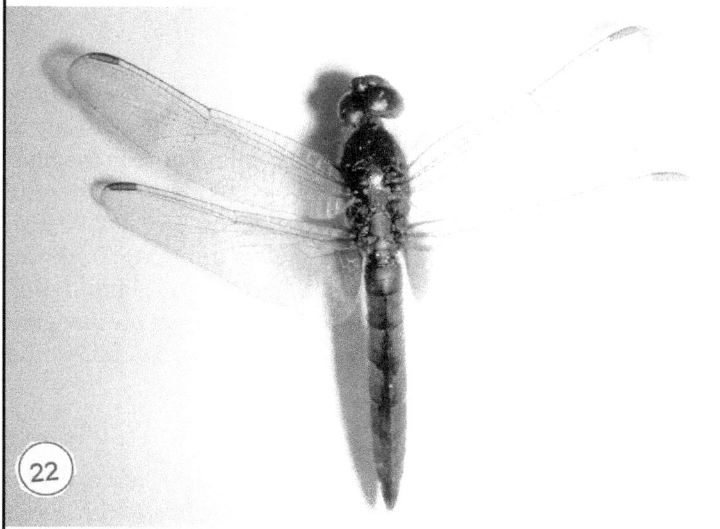

Figure 22: ***Trithemis pallidinervis*** **(Kirby); Male**

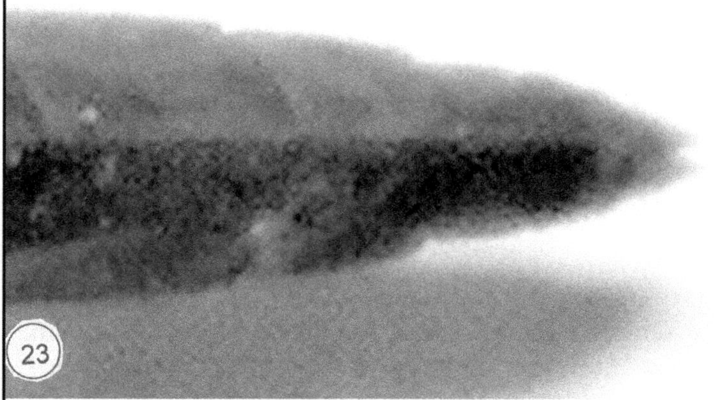

Figure 23: ***Trithemis pallidinervis:*** **Anal Appendages; Male**

3 lobed; anterior lobe 0.4 mm long, brown, middle lobe 5.3 mm long, 5.50 mm broad, olivaceous brown; posterior lobe 0.3 mm long, 5.50 mm broad; synthorax 7.00 mm long, 5.50 mm broad.

WINGS

Hyaline, with reddish reticulation and a bright ambur-yellow basal marking at extreme base in fore wing, but extending distally to first antenodal nervure and slightly over cubital nervure in the hind wing; pterostigma blackish with creamy white ends, membrane brown with attached border; Fore wing: 31.00 mm long, 7.00 mm broad, 65.00 mm wing span; pterostigma 2.90 mm long, 0.70 mm broad; antenodal nervures 12, postnodal neruvres 11; Hind wing: 29.00 mm long, 10.00 mm broad, 61.00 mm wing span; pterostigma 3.20 mm long, 0.74 mm broad; antenodal nervures 10½, postnodal nervure 10.

LEG

Hind leg 12.78 mm long 1.20 mm broad (width of coxa 1.20 mm); coxa 1.50 mm long, 1.20 mm broad, yellowish black with dense yellow hairs on inner side and outer side; trochanter 2 segmented; 1.40 mm long, 0.44 mm broad, blackish brown; 1st segment 0.40 mm long, 0.40 mm broad with blackish brown; 2nd segment 1.00 mm long, 0.44 mm broad, blackish brown with few yellow hairs on inner side and outer side; 0.42 mm part of trochanter overlaps on femora; femora 3.88 mm long, 0.40 mm broad; blackish brown with 11 spines on inner side; tibia 3.90 mm long, 0.22 mm broad; blackish brown with 11 pointed spines on inner side; tarsus 3 segmented, 1.60 mm long, 0.20 mm broad; 1st segment 0.36 mm long, 0.14 mm broad with two pointed spines on inner side. 2nd segment 0.74 mm long, 0.12 mm broad with 5 spines on inner side; 3rd segment 0.50 mm long, 0.20 mm broad with 4 spines on inner side; claw 0.50 mm long 0.18 mm broad with 4 spines.

ABDOMEN

24.00 mm long, 3.00 mm broad; long and slender, basal segments slightly tumid; black marked with bright reddish yellow. The sides of segments 1st to 3rd very broad, extending well up on to dorsum on 1st and 2nd segments but tapering to apical border on 3rd segment; long wedge shaped spots on segments 4th to 7th and a small basal sub-dorsal spot on 8th segment; remaining segments black. Anal appendages (Figure 23): reddish yellow at base, black apically; superior anal appendage 1.70 mm long, 0.46 mm broad, with row of robust spines on ventral border.

COLOUR

Reddish yellow: Abdomen.

Reddish brown: Compound eyes, frons

Brown: Anteclypeus, postclypeus, thorax.

Yellow: Labium.

Black: Labrum, mandible, antenna.

Yellowish black: Coxa.

HOLOTYPE: Male, India, Maharashtra, Coll. 3-X-2004; Koregaon, Satara district, M.S., Shinde, K.P., antenna, leg on slide labelled as above, other parts with pined form, labelled as above.

PARATYPE: Coll. 28-X-2004; same data as above.

DISTRIBUTIONAL RECORD/OBSERVATIONS

Male 17, Female 2. Sondari ♂1, 5-XII-2004; Maldeo ♂3, 19-XII-2004; Tapola ♂2, 2-I-2005; Khirkhindi ♂1; 6-III-2005; Dara ♂1, 8-V-2005; Zandoli ♂1, 22-V-2005; Jungti ♂3, 4-IX-2005; Kusawade ♂1♀1; Navaja ♂2, 6-X-2005; Kamargaon ♂2, 5-IV-2006.

GENUS *RHYOTHEMIS* HAGEN

The Genus *Rhyothemis* is erected by Hagen in 1867. This genus is distributed through out the tropical regions from Africa to Oceania. Under this genus five species have been reported from India. The species of this genus are gregarious and occur usually in large colonies over marshy spots or large weedy tanks in which they breed. Their flight is weak but often soaring and when flying low; the wing-action is fluttering like that of the larger Lepidoptera. The species like *R. triangularis*, mimic bees in their flight, and derive considerable protection from birds.

The genus *Rhyothemis* show following characters:

1. The dragonflies of this genus are metallic coloured and wings partly or wholly coloured black and golden-yellow or steely blue-black.

2. Head small, eyes broadly contiguous; frons rounded in both sexes, crest but slightly defined; vesicle large, broadly rounded.
3. Prothorax with small posterior lobe; thorax narrow small;
4. Legs long and slim; hind femora with rows of rather widely spaced, very small spines and a single longer one at distal end; similar in the sexes.
5. Wings variable, broad at base, pointed at apex, or long and moderately broad at base, varying in shape in the sexes of some species, where they are long and narrow in the male, short and very broad in the female; reticulation close; broadly marked with black and goden amber or with steely blue-black; discoidal cell in fore-wing rather narrow, its costal side about half the length of basal or distal, traversed once or more; discoidal cell in hind-wing with base at level of arc entire.
6. 7½ to 10½ antenodal nervures, distal one incomplete, 1 cubital nervure to all wings, subtrigone in fore-wing absent or many celled, pterostigma small, membrane large.
7. Abdomen relatively short, markedly compressed in both sexes.
8. Female with borders of segment 8 not dilated.

RHYOTHEMIS RANGINI SP.NOV.

MALE (Figures 24, 25)

29.00 mm in body length excluding anal appendages; head 30.00 mm long; thorax 8.00 mm long; fore wing 23.00 mm long, hind wing 22.00 mm long; abdomen 18.00 mm long, black with grayish tinge; superior anal appendages 1.10 mm long, yellow with black tip.

HEAD

3.00 mm long, 4.2 mm broad, roughly rounded, black; occiput black, hairy; compound eyes large, roughly circular, blackish brown, occular space 2.1 mm; 3 ocelli in triangle posterior one reddish brown at centre with basal yellow large ring; other two ocelli with blackish brown at centre and with basal yellow ring; posterior ocelli space 0.32 mm; interocellar space 0.72 mm; frons dark black, front with

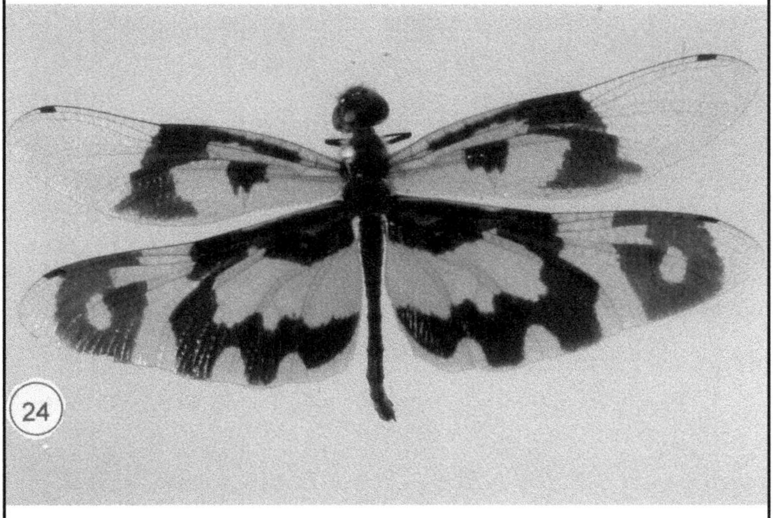

Figure 24: *Rhyothemis rangini* sp.nov.; Male

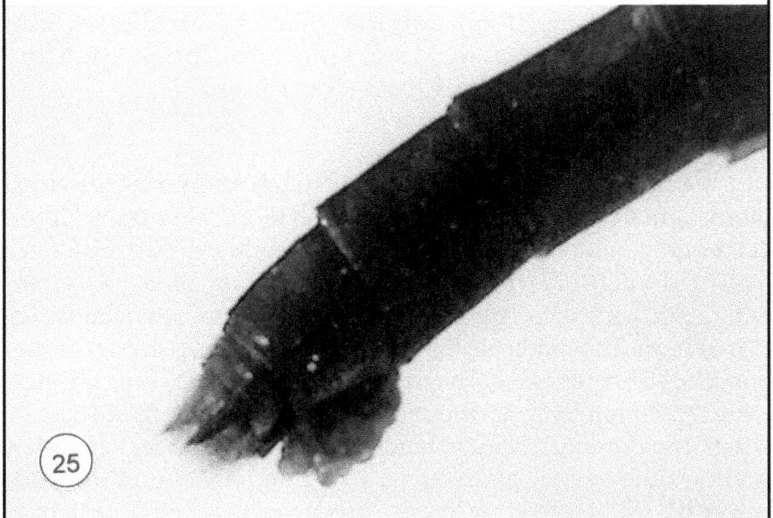

Figure 25: *Rhyothemis rangini:* Anal Appendages; Male

deep sulcus, scanty black hairs; postclypeus black; anteclypeus black with basal deep sulcus; labrum thick large, metalic greenishblue brown hairs; mandibles brown, mandible bases yellow, labium black with yellowish brown border.

Antenna

1.18 mm long, 0.12 mm broad (at scape); blackish brown with yellow rings, tip yellowish; interantennal space 1.16 mm; scape 0.6 mm long, 0.12 mm broad; Flagellum black, 5 segmented; 1st segment 0.22 mm long, 0.04 mm broad; 2nd segment 0.18 mm long, 0.035 mm broad; 3rd segment 0.20 mm long, 0.02 mm broad; 4th segment 0.16 mm long, 0.015 mm broad; 5th segment 0.16 mm long, 0.01 mm broad.

Flagellar Formula

L/W = ½ = 5.5/6; $^{2/2}$ = 6/6; $^{3/2}$ = 10/6; $^{4/2}$ = 10.6/6; $^{5/2}$ = 16/6; A = 1.59.

THORAX

8.00 mm long, 3.7 mm broad; black, not metallic green; prothorax 5.00 mm long, 3.7 mm broad; black not blackishbrown, 3 segmented; anterior lobe black, 0.7 mm long, 3.7 mm broad, hairy; mid lobe black, 4.00 mm long, 3.7 mm broad; prothorax with middorsal deep sulcus, posterior lobe 0.3 mm long, 4 mm broad, black; synthorax 3.00 mm long, 4.00 mm broad, black robust, broad.

WINGS

Wings hyaline at apices with black thick border upto pterostigma; base of wing deep brownish black; apex transparent, black venation, reticulation close, thick; Fore wing: narrow longer than hind wing; fore wing 23.00 mm long, 6.00 mm broad, 50.00 mm wing span; wings dark black brown extending more than mid area. Pterostigma 2.44 mm long, 0.66 mm broad, not reddish darkbrown but dark brown; antenodal nervures 9; post nodal nervures 14; Hind wing: 22.00 mm long, 8.5 mm broad, 47.00 mm wing span; base of wing deep brownish black extending more than mid region, rest of portion transparent; pterostigma 2.70 mm long, 1.8 mm broad, blackish brown with serrate border; antenodal nervures 9, postnodal nervures 11.

LEG

Hind leg 16.50 mm long, 1.8 mm broad, not entirely black but more or less reddish brown and black; coxa 1.70 mm long, 1.18 mm broad, blackish brown with yellow hairs, bunch of hairs internal and dense hairs outer side, hairs 0.32 mm long; trochanter 2 segmented, 1st segment 0.40 mm long, 0.36 mm broad, yellow; 2nd segment 0.70 mm long, 0.36 mm broad, yellow, no spines, only black mark on outer side; 0.22 mm part of femora covered by trochanter; femora 4.30 mm long, 0.36 mm broad, blackish brown, 34 small hairs on femora, 7 black thick, pointed, small spines with 0.14 mm length, only one large spine at basal region with 0.44 mm length, black, pointed; tibia 5.30 mm long, 0.16 mm broad, brown, 12 pair of long elongated, thin, pointed spines, spine 0.80 mm in length, six small sized spines on apical end of tibia, few yellowish hairs; tarsus 3 segmented; 1st segment 0.80 mm long, 0.36 mm broad with one spine; 2nd segment 0.80 mm long, 0.18 mm broad, brown, 4 spines; 3rd segment 0.90 mm long, 0.20 mm broad, brown, 4 spines; claws brownish black, 0.60 mm long, 0.18 mm broad, with yellow spines.

ABDOMEN

18.00 mm long, 1.8 mm broad, not entirely black but with greyish tinge, segments 1, 2, small black; segments 3, 4 broad, segments 6 to 9 on the mid with plate like structure, dorsal region, segment 10 small, segment 9th and 10th with basal region yellow, annulie on the border of 10th segment, black serrate margin. Anal appendages (Figure 25): 1.10 mm long, 0.2 mm broad, yellow, tip black; inferior anal appendages 0.90 mm long, 0.70 mm broad, brown with black tip and yellowish dense hairs.

COLOUR

Black: Abdomen, occiput, frons, thorax, labium

Yellow: Superior anal appendages

Blackish brown: ocelli, antenna.

Brown: Inferior anal appendages.

Metalic greenish blue: Labrum.

HOLOTYPE: Male, India, Maharashtra, Coll. 19-IX-2004 Kamargaon, Satara district, M.S., Shinde K.P., antenna, leg on slide labelled as above, other parts with pinned form, labelled as above.

PARATYPE: Male, Coll. 23-I-2005, same data as above.

DISTRIBUTIONAL RECORD/OBSERVATIONS

Male 7, Female 1. Mirgaon ♂1, ♀1, 3-X-2004; Patan ♂1, 26-XII-2004; Navaja ♂1, 3-IV-2005; Kusapur ♂2, 5-VI-2005; Yerad ♂2, 13-XI-2005.

DISCUSSION

This species runs close to *Rhyothemis triangularis* Kirby by having following characters.

1. Wing bases deep brownish black.
2. Apices of wings hyaline.
3. Pterostigma small.

However, it differs from above species by following characters.

1. Prothorax black
2. Abdomen black with greyish tinge
3. Pterostigma dark brownish, not dark reddish brown.
4. Abdominal appendages not entirely black, superior yellow with black tip; inferior brown with black tip.
5. Legs not entirely black, trochanter yellow. Coxa blackish brown, femora blackish brown, tibia brown, claws blackish brown.
6. Fore wing–Antenodal nervures 9, postnodal nervures 14. Hind wing–Antenodal nervures 9, post nodal nervures 11.
7. Flagellar Formula: L/W = ½ = 5.5/6; $^{2/2}$ = 6/6; $^{3/2}$ = 10/6; $^{4/2}$ = 10.6/6; $^{5/2}$ = 16/6; A = 1.59.

GENUS *GYNACANTHA* RAMBUR

This genus was erected by Rambur in 1842. The genus is distributed throughout the world, but confined to the tropical and non-tropical zones. Out of fifty species known half of them are reported from the Oriental and Papuan regions, out of these, fourteen have been reported from India. With rare exceptions, all species are corespuscular by nature. Their principal food appears to be mosquitoes and microlepidoptera. During the day they may be flushed from dark thickets, especially bamboo in swampy low-lying country. These can be seized quite easily by the abdomen with the thumb and forefinger, an easy way of catching them. The female deposits her eggs in dry soil in gullies sloping down to swamps. In these spots the ova probably lie until the next rain, when freshet washes down into swamp below. During oviposition the female invariably off her long cylinder anal appendages. The adult insects are often very beautiful in their display of blended greens and blues. The genus is further characterised by:

1. Large size, colouring of dull brown and greens.
2. Head large and globular.
3. Eyes very broadly contiguous.
4. Occiput nearly obsolete
5. Thorax comparatively small
6. Legs rather short; hind femora armed with two rows of short closely set spines.
7. Wings long and broad, very closely reticulated.
8. Pterostigma moderately long, very narrow.
9. 6 to 10 cubital nervures in all wings, no incomplete basal antenodal nervures present.
10. Anal appendages very long, very narrow; and coated with long hairs on the inner side of apical half.
11. Inferior appendage narrowly triangular, not emarginate.
12. Segment 10 prolonged laterally and ventrally into a long two-prolonged plate, the curved prongs or spines strongly divaricate.

Gynacantha Rambur, Ins. Nevrop. p. 209 (1842); Selys, in Sagrals Hist. cuba, Ins. p. 459 (1857); Hagen, Neur. N. Amer. p. 131 (1861); Kirby, Cat. Odon. p. 94 (1890); Karsch, Ent. Nachr. vol. xvii, p. 276 (1891); Kruger, Stett. Ent. Zeit. vol. lix, pp. 307-311 (1898); Martin, Cat., Coll. Selys (Aeschnines), fase, xx, pp. 8, 167 (1909); Ris, Ann. Soc. Ent, Belg. Vol. iv, pp. 244, 245 (1911); id., Nova Guinea, xiii, livr, Z. Zool, pp. 106, 107 (1915); id., Ann. S. African Mus. vol. xviii, p. 357 (1920); Laidlaw, Rec. Ind. Mus. vol. xxii, p. 90 (1921); Fraser, J. Bombay Nat. Hist. Soc. vol. xxviii, pp. 111, 902, 903 (1922); Laidlaw, Proc. U.S. Nat. Mus. vol. lxii, pp. 19, 20, 27 (1923); Williamson, Miscellan Publications Mus. Zool. Univ. Michigan, No. 9, pp. 4-7

(1923); Laidlaw, J. F. M. S. Mus. vol. xvi, p. 177 (1930); Needham, Zool. Sinica, Ser. A, vol. xi, p. 88, (1930); id., Rec. Ind. Mus. vol. xxxiv, p. 216 (1932).

GYNACANTHA SATHEI SP.NOV.

MALE (Figures 26, 27)

70.00 mm body length excluding anal appendages, head 7.00 mm long, thorax 13.00 mm long, fore wing 49.00 mm long, hind wing 50.00 mm long, abdomen 50.00 mm long; superior anal appendages 6.00 mm long, brown with black tip.

HEAD

Large, globular, 7.00 mm long, 9.00 mm broad, roughly triangular; occiput nearly obsolete yellow; compound eyes very broadly contiguous, bluish with black spots; occular space 3.5 mm; three ocelli in triangle, brown at centre, ocelli base with yellow ring, ocellar space 0.30 mm; interocellar space 0.72 mm; frons yellowish green with 'T' shaped thick black markings; postclypeus greenish yellow; anteclypeus yellow; labrum yellowish brown; mandibles black, bases of mandibles brown; labium brown not yellowish.

Antenna

7 segmented, brown with yellow rings, 2.28 mm long, 0.30 mm broad (width of scape 0.30 mm); interantennal space 1.30 mm; scape 0.10 mm long, 0.30 mm broad; pedicel 0.3 mm long, 0.22 mm broad. Flagellum: 5 segmented, 1.88 mm long, 0.04 mm broad; 1st segment 0.40 mm long, 0.04 mm broad; 2nd segment 0.20 mm long, 0.032 mm broad; 3rd segment 0.22 mm long, 0.024 mm broad; 4th segment 0.30 mm long, 0.015 mm broad; 5th segment 0.76 mm long, 0.01 mm broad.

Flagellar Formula

L/W; ½ = 10/6.25; $^{2/2}$ = 6.25/6.25; $^{3/2}$ = 9.16/6.25; $^{4/2}$ = 20/6.25; $^{5/2}$ = 76/6.25; A = 3.88.

THORAX

13.00 mm long, 7.00 mm broad; without two sharply defined blackish brown stripes on each side, yellowish hairy; without reddish brown on dorsum, 7.00 mm long, 7.00 mm broad, brown with yellow hairs at dorsal side, on mid dorsal region one black plate; prothorax yellowish brown, with blackish median stripe, 3

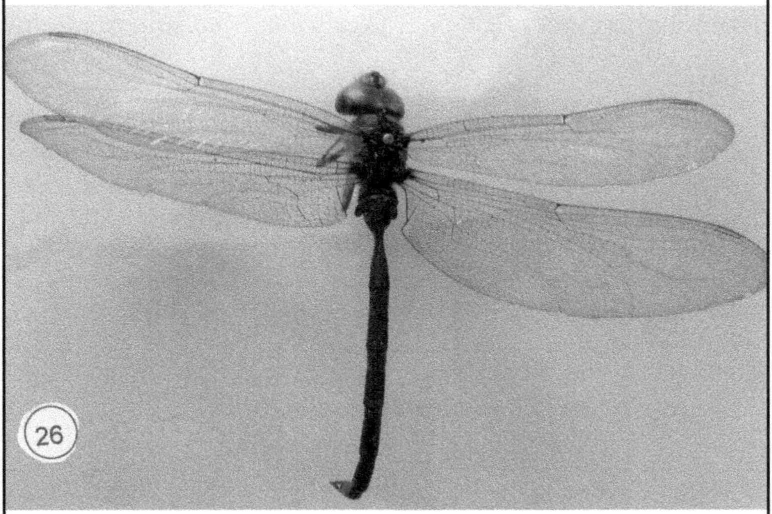

Figure 26: *Gynacantha sathei* sp.nov.; Male

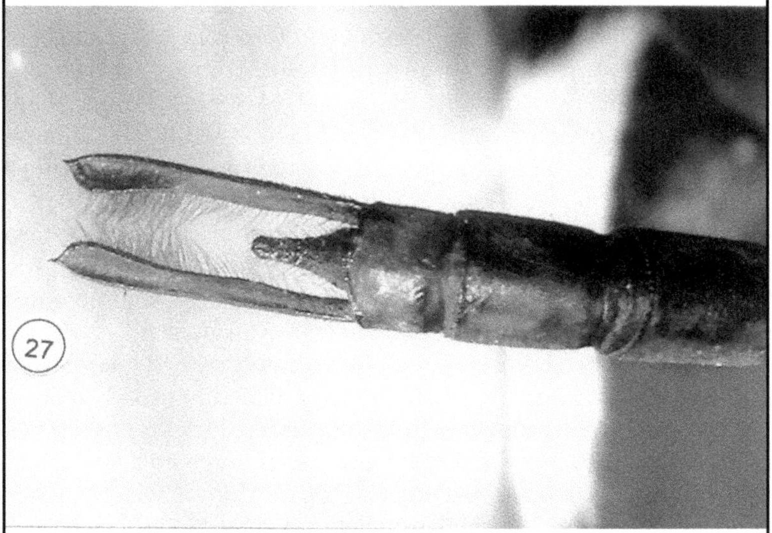

Figure 27: *Gynacantha sathei:* Anal Appendages; Male

lobed, anterior lobe 0.7 mm long, middle lobe 6.00 mm long, posterior lobe 0.3 mm long, brown; synthorax 6.00 mm long, 7.00 mm broad, rough, dorsolaterally yellowish with very thin, black stripes laterally.

WINGS

Wing apices bordered with dark yellowish brown but not with blackish brown, 2 cells from costal line; wings hyaline, costal border dark yellowish; reticulation close, yellowish brown venation, wing bases dark brownish black, transparent. Fore wing: 49.00 mm long, 11.00 mm broad, 102.00 mm wing span; pterostigma 3.10 mm long, 0.70 mm broad, half red and half yellow; antenodal nervures 28, postnodal nervures 22. Hind wing: large, 50.00 mm, 14.00 mm broad, 104.00 mm wing span, pterostigma 2.70 mm long, 0.78 mm broad, yellow, inner side black; outer costal side red with black spots; antenodal nervures 21, postnodal nervures 25.

LEG

Hind leg 21.70 mm long, 1.80 mm broad, (coxa diameter 1.80 mm), red and yellow with black spines and yellow hairs; coxa 1.70 mm long, 1.80 mm broad, yellow with yellowish white long hairs on inner side and bunch of yellowish white hairs on outer side. Trochanter 2 segmented, 1.90 mm long, 0.76 mm broad, red; 1st segment 0.40 mm long, 0.76 mm broad, reddish brown with yellow dense hairs on inner side; 2nd segment 1.50 mm long, 0.76 mm broad, 0.80 mm part overlaps on femora, reddish brown, with 2 yellow hairs and only two black pointed spines on inner side, no spines and hairs on outer side; femora 7.00 mm long, 0.70 mm broad, red, outerside near trochanter only two small, thin, blackish spines; spines 0.18 mm long, on posterior side one yellow long spine, spine 0.34 mm long, a row of small black, thick, pointed spines on outer side; many small, black, thick, pointed spines on inner side; reddish, long, thin, pointed hairs and blackish brown spines on lateral side. Spines 0.38 mm long; tibia 7.80 mm long, 0.50 mm broad, yellow, tibia base and apex reddish with 13 pairs of red thick pointed spines inner side and 10 pairs of thin yellow spines outer side, spine 0.30 mm long; tarsus two segmented, red, 2.50 mm long, 0.26 mm broad; 1st segment 1.20 mm long, 0.26 mm broad, red with 6 reddish brown spines; 2nd segment 1.30 mm long, 0.18 mm broad, red with 5 reddish brown spines; claws 0.80 mm long, 0.20 mm broad, dark red with two long and two small spines.

ABDOMEN

Large, 50.00 mm long, 5.00 mm broad; 1st and 2nd abdominal segments very tumid at base, 3rd segment markedly constricted at mid basally, broad, bluish green; on 2nd segment bluishgreen flaps, each segment black apically and with greenish yellow bands basally. Segments 4th to 8th long, at basal region with double serrate margin. Segment 9 and 10 yellowish. Anal appendages (Figure 27): not thick at base but narrower than tip; superior anal appendages 6.00 mm long, 0.70 mm broad, blackish brown with black tip and dense yellowish hairs from inner side; inferior anal appendages 1.4 mm long, 0.68 mm broad, less than half the length of superior, triangular, brown.

COLOUR

Yellow: Occiput, frons, postclypeus, anteclypeus.

Brown: Anal appendages, labium, antenna, inferior anal appendages; thorax.

Bluish green: 1st and 2nd abdominal segments.

Black: mandible

Blackish brown: Labrum, superior anal appendages.

HOLOTYPE: Male, India, Maharashtra, Coll. 7-XI-2004; Kusawade, Satara district, M.S., Shinde K.P., antenna, leg on slide, labelled as above, other parts with pined form, labelled as above.

PARATYPE: Male 1, Coll. 19-XII-2004, same data as above.

DISTRIBUTIONAL RECORD/OBSERVATIONS

Male 11; female 1. Morgiri ♂1, 20-IV-2005; Nisare ♂ 2, 13-VI-2005; Sondari ♂2, 20-XII-2005; Munawale ♂2, 15-I-2006; Tapola ♂ 2, ♀1, 6-III-2006; Maldeo ♂1, 21-V-2006.

DISCUSSION

This species runs close to *Gynacantha basiguttata* Selys by having following characters:

1. Wings not tipped with dark brown.
2. Abdomen and wings more than 45 and 40 mm respectively.
3. Eyes bluish with black spots.

However, it differ from above species by having following characters:

1. Labrum yellowish brown.
2. Labium brown, not yellowish.
3. Thorax yellowish without definate brown stripes.
4. Prothorax with blackish median stripe on dorsal side.
5. Wing tips not with blackish brown.
6. Pterostigma half yellow and half red.
7. Legs not entirely reddish brown, tibia not black.
8. Flagellar Formula: L/W; ½ = 10/6.25; $^{2/2}$ = 6.25/6.25; $^{3/2}$ = 9.16/6.25; $^{4/2}$ = 20/6.25; $^{5/2}$ = 76/6.25; A = 3.88.
9. Anal appendages not thick at base but narrower than it's tip.
10. 1st and 2nd abdominal segments bluish green.

GENUS *ANAX* LEACH

The genus *Anax* was raised by Leach in 1815. The genus is cosmopolitant in distribution. Five species of this genus have been reported from India. Out of which two are confined in montane and three in plain regions of India. All breed in small weedy tanks and lakes except *A. immaculifrons,* which is riverine in habitat. They are familiar insects on all open waters, and may be seen ceaselessly and restlessly hawking round and round the borders of tanks. The male accompanies the female during the action of oviposition, keeping off intruders and those of it's own species. *A. immaculifrons,* although the most feral species of the genus, during the dry months will leave its jungly habitats and take to the surrounding plains. They are among the largest and most robust dragonflies of the Indian fauna.

Genus shows following characters:

1. Dragonflies of very large size and robust build, variably coloured.
2. Wings hyaline, but often partly tinted with yellow or pale brown.
3. Head very large, globular; eyes broadly contiguous,
4. Frons with sharply angled fore-border or crest but not elevated.

5. Occiput very small.
6. Thorax robust.
7. Legs long and robust, femora armed with rows of short, closely set spines and with two or three longer ones at distal end.
8. Wings long and broad, apices pointed, base straight, reticulation close; discoidal cells very elongate, very narrow, that of fore wing more so than the hind, made up of 3 to 7 cells, usually 6 in fore-wing and 5 in the hind.
9. Abdomen tumid at base, often slightly constricted at segment 3, then cylindrical or slightly depressed at end segments.
10. Anal appendages: superiors very homogeneous in the genus, broadly lanceolate, bluntly rounded at apices, with a small spine on the outer side of apex and a very strong ridge on upper surface; inner upper surface towards apex, coated with long hairs, inferior appendage quadrate.

Anax imperator Leech, Edinb. Encycl. vol. ix p. 137 (1815); Kirby, Cat. odon. pp. 84, 85 (1890); Lucas, Brit. Dragonflies, pp. 163-170, pl. xii, Figure 34 (1900): Tillyard, Biology of Dragonflies, pp. 341, 342, Figure 172 (1917); Morton., Ent. Month, Mag.; (3) Vol. vi, p. 85 (1920); Schmidt, Die Tierwelt Mitteleuropas, vol. iv, 7 ordnung, Libellen, p. 40 (1929); Lucas, Aquatic Stage of Brit. Dragonflies (larva) pp. 56-58, Pl. X (1930).

Aeshna formosa Lind., Opuse. Scient. vol. iv, p. 158, t. 4, Figure 1 (1823); id., Mon. Lib. Eur. p. 20 (1825); Fonscolomb, Ann. Soc. Ent.; France, vol. vii, p.; 79, t. T, Figure 1 (1838).

Aeschna azurea Charpentier, Horae Ent. p. 31 (1825); id., Lit. Eur. p. 99, t. 17 and t. 45, Figure 1 (1840).

Anax formosa Stephens, III Brit. Ent., Mana, vol. vi, p. 81 (1836); Selys, Mon. Lib. Eur. p. 117 (1840).

Aeschna (Anax) formosa Selys, Bull. Acad. Belg. (2) vol. vi, p. 387 (1839).

Anax formosa Rambur, Ins. Nevrop. p. 182, t. 1, Figure 12 (1842); Selys, Rev. Odon. p. 110 (1850); Brauer Reise and Novara, Neur, p. 60 (1866); Hagen, Verh. Zool. bot. Ges., Wien, vol. xvii, p. 48 (1867); Martin, Cat. Coll. Selys. fase, xviii, pp. 9, 10 Figure 2 (1908).

ANAX MAHALAXMI SP. NOV.

MALE (Figures 28, 29)

72.00 mm body length excluding anal appendages, head 7.00 mm long, thorax 14.00 mm long, fore wing 55.00 mm long, hind wing 51.00 mm long; abdomen 51.00 mm long, black with yellowish and blue bands, superior anal appendages 6.00 mm long, 1.1 mm broad, blackish brown, hairy.

HEAD

7.00 mm long, 10.00 mm broad, roughly rounded; occiput yellow; eyes broadly contiguous, blackish brown; occular space 3.5 mm; three ocelli in triangle, anterior ocelli yellow, ocellar space 0.30 mm; posterior two ocelli brown with basal yellow ring, interocellar space 1.04 mm; frons bluish green with red line; bordered by yellowish colouration; postclypeus yellowish green, anteclypeus greenish with two brown spots; labrum yellow; mandibles black, mandible bases pale greenish; Labium brown; labium mid lobe black; lateral lobe yellowish brown.

ANTENNA

2.74 mm long, 0.24 mm broad, 7 segmented, black; scape 0.06 mm long (width of scape 0.24 mm), 0.24 mm broad; pedicel 0.52 mm long, 0.22 mm broad; Flagellum: 5 segmented, 2.16 mm long; 0.08 mm broad; 1st segment 0.80 mm long, 0.08 mm broad; 2nd segment 0.32 mm long, 0.06 mm broad; 3rd segment 0.38 mm long, 0.39 mm broad; 4th segment 0.28 mm long, 0.19 mm broad; 5th segment 0.38 mm long, 0.009 mm broad.

Flagellar Formula

L/W: ½ = 10/5.33; $^{2/2}$ = 5.33/5.33; $^{3/2}$ = 9.74/5.33; $^{4/2}$ = 14.73/ 5.33; $^{5/2}$ = 42.22/5.33; A = 2.92.

THORAX

14.00 mm long, 9.00 mm broad; robust grayish black with yellow hairs and bluish shed on dorsal side; blue and black bands on lateral sides; prothorax 9.00 mm long, 8.00 mm broad; 3 lobed, anterior lobe 0.9 mm long, blackish with yellowish hairs, anterior colour yellow; mid lobe 6.8 mm long, 8.00 mm broad, yellowish with yellow hairs and blue shed dorsolaterally; posterior lobe plate like, 0.3 mm long,

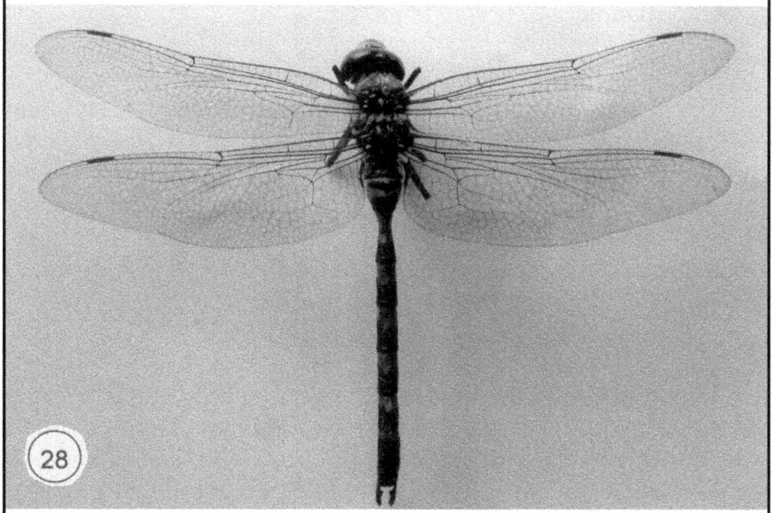

Figure 28: *Anax mahalaxmi* sp.nov.; Male

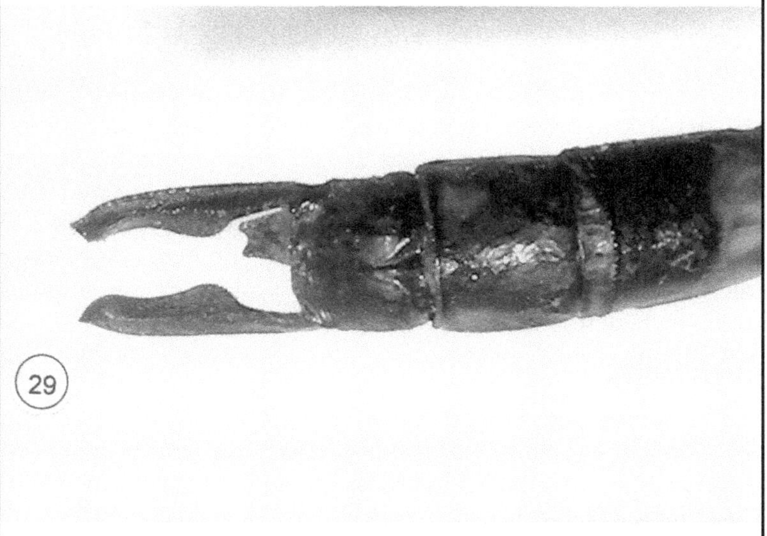

Figure 29: *Anax mahalaxmi:* Anal Appendages; Male

8.00 mm broad; synthorax 5.00 mm long, 8.00 mm broad; robust dorsally blackish brown with blue plates and laterally two blue and two black bands.

WINGS

Wings long and broad, apices pointed, base straight; reticulation close; wings hyaline wings tinted yellow except some basal portion. Fore wing: 55.00 mm long, 12.00 mm broad, wing span 114.00 mm; pterostigma 3.7 mm long, 0.70 mm broad, brown; antenodal nervures 19, postnodal nervures 9. Hind wing: 51.00 mm long, 15.00 mm broad, 105 mm wing span; pterostigma 4.4 mm long, 0.60 mm broad, brown, antenodal nervures 14, postnodal nervures 12.

LEG

Hind leg 30.96 mm long, 2.60 mm broad (width of coxa 2.60 mm), black with hairs and spines; coxa 1.90 mm, 2.60 mm broad with bunch of yellow dense hairs on inner side; trochanter two segmented, 2.74 mm long 1.00 mm broad, black; 1st segment 0.96 mm long, 1.00 mm broad, black with bunch of hairs on posterior side; 2nd segment 1.78 mm long, 1.00 mm broad, black with only 4 yellow hairs on inner side; 0.26 mm part covers femora; femora 11.20 mm long, 0.94 mm broad, black with thick, black pointed spines on inner side, spines downwardly directed, only last spine long; last spines long, femora 0.30 mm long, also with yellow hairs and small black thick, pointed spines on outer side; tibia 10.00 mm long, 0.56 mm broad, blackish brown, on inner side 11 black, thick, blunt spines, spine 0.8 mm long; tarsus 2 segmented; 2.74 mm in length, 0.40 mm broad, reddish brown; tarsus 2 segmented; 1st segment 1.68 mm long, 0.40 mm broad with 5 black, thick, pointed spines; 2nd segment 2.10 mm long, 0.34 mm broad with 5 black, thick, pointed spines inner side; claws 1.34 mm long, 0.22 mm broad with 4 spines, two spines large, thick, reddish brown and 2 spines small red.

ABDOMEN

51.00 mm long, 6.00 mm broad; reddish brown with blue and black bands; segment 1st 6.00 mm broad, blue with black spots; segment 2nd narrow, 3.00 mm broad, brown with black band; 3rd to 8th segment, 4.00 mm broad, brown with black bands; segment 1st to 7th middorsal black narrow plate, segment 9th and 10th black; superior and appendages 6.00 mm long, 1.10 mm broad with brown basal part. Anal appendages (Figure 29): not reddish brown, black anterior part, superior anal appendages flat with black dense hairy; inferior 3.5 mm long, 1.04 mm broad, quadrate in shape, yellow with black tip, inferior less than half the length of superior touching to widest part of superior.

GENUS *PANTALA* HAGEN

The Genus *Pantala* was erected by Hagen in 1861. This is cosmopolitan genus and widely distributed throughout the tropical and subtropical zones of the old and new worlds. This dominant genus contains only two species, one of which has encircled the world in its distribution. The dragonflies of this genus breed in marshes and weedy shallow lakes and emerge in millions during the month of September to start a steady and sustained migration which may go in for some weeks (in the case of *P. flaviscens* this migratory flight is an annual event and goes on continuously throughout September and October). Only this latter species is found within our limits.

This genus shows following characters.

1. The dragonflies are rather large sized and robust build, coloured ochreous or reddish and with uncoloured wings.
2. Head large, eyes rather broadly contiguous.
3. Frons broad and projecting and presenting two oval flat surfaces anteriorly separated by a deep sulcus.
4. Vesicle broad and depressed.
5. Prothorax with very small posterior lobe; thorax robust.
6. Legs slim, moderately long; hind femora with numerous closely set, evenly sized spines, these are in the proximal two thirds; wider spaced and longer spines in the distal third.
7. Abdomen robust, dilated at basal segments, slightly constricted at segment 3, then gradually tapered to the end.
8. Wings long and broad, especially at base, narrow and pointed at apices, reticulation close.
9. In the fore wing discoidal cell is traversed, with costal side hardly one-third the length of basal or distal sides; that of hind wing with base at level of arc, entire;

10. Sectors of arc widely fused in all wings; arc situated between the first and second antenodal nervures; about 13½ antenodal nervures the distal one incomplete.
11. I cubital nervure in fore-wing, 2 in the hind; discoidal field in fore-wing with 3 rows of cells at beginning, its borders converging strongly at wing border; no supplementary nervure to bridge.
12. Subtrigone in fore-wing 3 or 4 celled; 2 rows of cells between IRiii and RSpl;
13. Anal loop long and slim, distal side not markedly angled and the angle very obtuse, its apex closed.
14. Pterostigma small, pterostigma of hind wing distinctly smaller than the fore wing; membrane moderately large.

Pantala Hagen, Syn. Neur. Amer. p. 141 (1861); Brauer, Verh. Zool. bot. Ges. Wien, vol. xviii, pp. 364, 713 (1868); Mac Lachlan, Proc. Zool. Soc. Lond. vol. xii, pp 258, 265 (1889); id; cat. Odon. p. 2 (1890); Calvert, Proc. Calif. Acad. (2) Vol. iv, p. 471 (1895); id., Biol. C. Amer., Neur. pp. 203, 307 (1905-1906); Forster, Jber. Mannheim. vols. lxxi, lxxii, p. 4 (Sep.) (1906); Ris, Cat. Coll. Selys, Fascs, ix, xv, pp 34, 915-917 (1909-1913); Fraser, J. Bombay Nat. Hist. Soc. vol. xxvii pp. 49, 50 (1920).

PANTALA FLAVESCENS FABRICIUS

MALE (Figures 30, 31)

46.00 mm body length excluding anal appendages, head 6.00 mm long; thorax 10.00 mm long, fore wing 45.00 mm long, hind wing 41.00 mm long, abdomen 30.00 mm long; superior anal appendages 2.96 mm long, reddish brown with black tip.

HEAD

6.00 mm long, 7.00 mm broad, roughly rounded; occiput yellow; compound eye reddish brown, broadly contiguous; occular space 3.00 mm, ocellar space 0.22 mm; interocellar space 1.80 mm; frons broad and projecting and presenting two oval flat surfaces anteriorly separated by a deep sulcus, yellow reddish in front; postclypeus yellow, anteclypeus yellow; labrum brown, not border by black; mandibles black; labium mid lobe black and lateral lobe brown with dense hairs not yellowish.

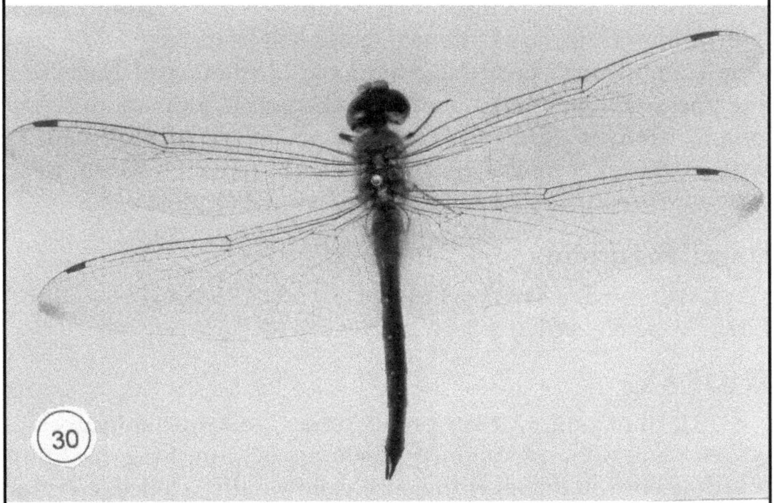

Figure 30: *Pantala flavescens* Fabricius; Male

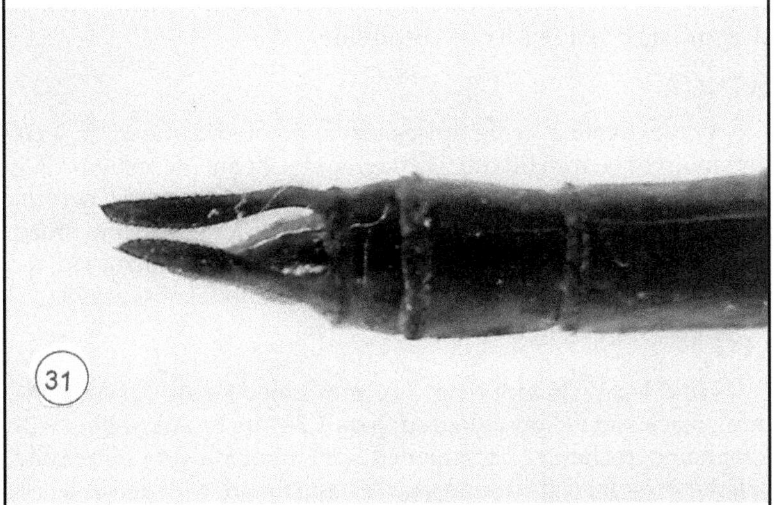

Figure 31: *Pantala flavescens:* Anal Appendages; Male

Antenna

1.88 mm long, 0.18 mm broad (width of scape 0.18 mm), black with yellow rings; interantennal space 1.46 mm; scape 0.06 mm long, 0.18 mm broad; pedicel 0.38 mm long, 0.16 mm broad. Flagellum: 5 segmented, 1.44 mm long, 0.06 mm broad; 1st segment 0.48 mm long, 0.06 mm broad; 2nd segment 0.18 mm long, 0.39 mm broad; 3rd segment 0.32 mm long, 0.24 mm broad; 4th segment 0.16 mm long, 0.015 mm broad; 5th segment 0.30 mm long, 0.007 mm broad.

Flagellar Formula

L/W; ½ = 8/4.61; $^{2/2}$ = 4.61/4.61; $^{3/2}$ = 13.33/4.61; $^{4/2}$ = 10.66/ 4.61; $^{5/2}$ = 42.85/4.61 A = 3.44.

THORAX

10.00 mm long, 6.00 mm broad; robust; yellowish dorsally late yellow ventrally and laterally; prothorax 5.3 mm long, 6.00 mm broad, yellow on dorsal with dense yellow hairs; 3 lobed, anterior lobe 0.7 mm long, reddish brown; mid lobe 4.3 mm long, 6.00 mm broad, yellow with dense yellow hairs; posterior lobe 0.3 mm long, 6.00 mm broad, yellow dorsally with black shed, ventrally pale yellow; synthorax 4.00 mm long, 6.00 mm broad, robust, yellow on dorsal side and pale yellowish on ventral side.

WINGS

Wings hyaline, wing apices black, pointed; Fore wing: 45.00 mm long, 10.00 mm broad; 93.00 mm wing span; pterostigma 2.56 mm long, 0.62 mm broad, red with black margin; antenodal nervure 15, post nodal nervure 8; Hind wing: 41.00 mm long, 0.28 mm broad, 85.00 mm wing span; pterostigma 2.50 mm long, 0.66 mm broad, red with black border; antenodal nervure 8, post nodal nervures 9.

LEG

Hind leg 17.36 mm long, 1.02 mm broad (width of coxa 1.02 mm); black and yellow coloured; coxa 1.24 mm broad, yellow with long hairs; trochanter 2 segmented, 1.80 mm long, 0.44 mm broad, yellow; 1st segment 0.60 mm long, 0.44 mm broad, with dense yellow hairs on inner side; 2nd segment 1.20 mm long, 0.44 mm broad, yellow with yellow hairs on inner side; 0.70 mm part of trochanter overlaps on femora; femora 6.10 mm long, 0.40 mm broad, black with yellow strip with 17 spines; tibia 5.60 mm long, 0.20 mm broad, black with

20 black pairs of thin pointed spines, spines 0.50 mm long; tarsus 3 segmented, black; 1st segment 1.02 mm long, 0.16 mm broad, black, 10 spines black, on inner side, spine 0.28 mm long; 2nd segment 1.00 mm long, 0.16 mm broad, black with 6 spines black, thin, pointed on inner side, spine 0.24 mm long; 3rd segment, black with 5 black spines on inner side; claws 0.16 mm long, 0.12 mm broad, with reddish brown.

ABDOMEN

30.00 mm long, 3.00 mm broad; 1st to 4th segment yellow with reddish shed on dorsal side; segment 5th and 6th reddish with faint black strip on dorsal side; segment 7 to 10 reddish with dark black stripe on dorsal side. Anal appendages (Figure 31): brownish blackish; superior anal appendages 2.96 mm long, 0.26 mm broad, black with dense hairs on inner and outer side; inferior anal appendages 0.75 mm long, triangular, black.

COLOUR

Yellow: Occiput, frons, anteclypeus, postclypeus, thorax, coxa.

Black: Ocelli, mandible, antenna, superior anal appendages, tibia.

Brown: Labrum.

PREY RECORD: Pyralid moth, mosquitoes, jassids.

HOLOTYPE: Male, India, Maharashtra, Coll. 2, 10-X-2004; Kadoli, Satara district, M.S., Shinde K.P., antenna, leg on slide labelled as above, other parts with pined form, labelled as above.

PARATYPE: Male 1, Coll. 5-XII-2004, same data as above.

DISTRIBUTIONAL RECORD/OBSERVATIONS

Male 27, female 2; Ghatmatha ♂3, 26-IX-2004; Tapola ♂ 3, 7-XI-2004; Patan ♂4, ♀1, 21-XI-2004; Munawale ♂3, 19-XI-2004; Urul ♂3, 30-I-2005; Dara ♂4, 20-III-2005; Kamargaon ♂2, 8-V-2005; Ghanbi ♂2, ♀1, 10-VII-2005, Jungti ♂2, 12-II-2006; Zadoli ♂1, 21-V-2006.

PANTALA SHIVAJIENSIS SP.NOV.

MALE (Figures 32, 33)

45.00 mm in body length excluding anal appendages; head 5.00 mm long, thorax 12.00 mm long, fore wing 43.00 mm long, hind

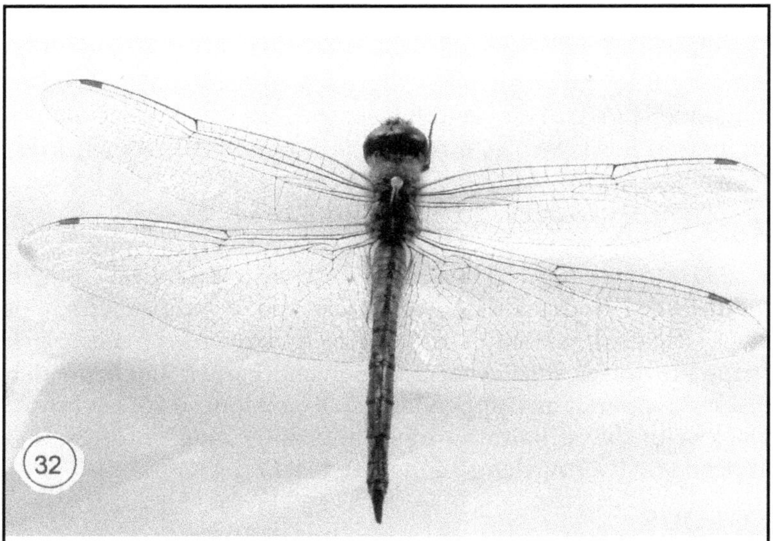
Figure 32: *Pantala shivajiensis* sp.nov.; Male

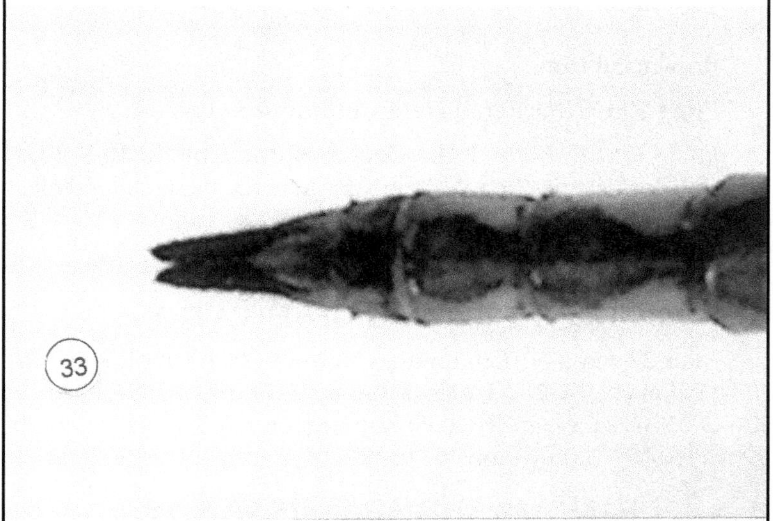
Figure 33: *Pantala shivajiensis:* Anal Appendages; Male

wing 40.00 mm long, abdomen 28.00 mm long, yellow with black patches, superior anal appendages 3.2 mm long with black except yellow basally with dense hairs.

HEAD

5.00 mm long, 8.00 mm broad, roughly circular, occiput yellow, compound eyes blackish brown, ocular space 4.00 mm; three ocelli in triangle, black, ocellar space 0.18 mm, introcellar space 1.40 mm; frons yellow with deep sulcus; postclypeus yellow, anteclypeus olivaceous yellow; labrum brown, mandible black; mandible bases brown, labium yellowish with middle lobe brown, border dark brown, lateral lobes brown.

Antenna

2.08 mm long, 0.15 mm broad (width of scape 0.15 mm); 7 segmented; scape 0.08 mm long, 0.22 mm broad; pedicel 0.20 mm long, 0.14 mm broad. Flagellum: 5 segmented, 1.80 mm long, 0.05 mm broad; 1st segment 0.40 mm long, 0.05 mm broad; 2nd segment 0.20 mm long, 0.041mm broad; 3rd segment 0.50 mm long, 0.017 mm broad; 4th segment 0.40 mm long, 0.014 mm broad; 5th segment 0.30 mm long, 0.009 mm broad.

Flagellar Formula

L/W; ½ = 8/4.87; $^{2/2}$ = 4.87/4.87; $^{3/2}$ = 29.41/4.87; $^{4/2}$ = 28.57/ 4.87; $^{5/2}$ = 33.3/4.87; A = 4.28.

THORAX

12.00 mm long, 6.00 mm broad, dull yellowish with dense yellowish downy hairs; prothorax 7.00 mm long, 6.00 mm broad, yellowish with dense yellowish hairs and one yellow transverse line dorsally and greenish patch laterally, 3 lobed; anterior lobe 0.5 mm long, black with hairs; middle lobe 6.2 mm long, 6.00 mm broad, dull yellowish with yellow hairs on dorsal and lateral side; anterior lobe with transverse yellow line on anterodorsal side and bluish patch on lateral side; posterier lobe 0.3 mm long, 6.00 mm broad yellowish with not transverse belt of dark and reddish brown between anterior and middle lobe; synthorax 5.00 mm long, 6.00 mm broad, yellow on dorsal side and bluish on lateral side, laterally no stripes on pro and synthorax.

WINGS (Figure 32)

Wings hyaline, wing apices brown and pointed, wing bases yellowish and on apical part of hind wing yellow patch; reticulation close, brownish reddish venation. Fore wing: 43.00 mm long 10.00 mm broad, 83.00 mm wing span; pterostigma 2.40 mm long, 0.60 mm broad, reddish pterostigma longer than in hind wing, antenodal nervures 16, postnodal nervures 8; fore wing with bluish tinge; Hind wing: 40.00 mm long, 16.00 mm broad, 89.00 mm wing span; pterostigma 2.40 mm long, 0.64 mm broad, reddish, antenodal nervures 8, postnodal nervures 10, on the apical region of hind wing yellow patch, apices acutely pointed and with brown spot and wings with bluish tinge, apical line of discoidal cell with three nervures and not 2½ nervures.

LEG

Hind leg 16.70 mm in length, 1.20 mm broad (width of coxa 1.20 mm), coxa 2.00 mm long, 1.20 mm broad, yellow reddish and whitish patch on outer side; trochanter 2 segmented; 1.70 mm long, 0.52 mm broad; 1st segment 0.60 mm long, 0.48 mm broad; whitish; 2nd segment 1.10 mm long, 0.52 mm broad with inner side whitish and outer side reddish; 0.40 mm part of trochanter overlaps on femora; femora 5.90 mm in length, 0.38 mm broad, anterior half part yellowish and posterior half part blackish with anterior side one black transverse ring and inner side 20 black pointed thick spines, length of spine 0.30 mm and 11 yellow thin spines on inner side, length of yellow spine 0.42 mm; tibia 4.60 mm long, 0.20 mm broad, black with 24 long, thin reddish spines on inner side and 20 very small black pointed spines on outer side; tarsus 3 segmented, 2.50 mm long, 0.20 mm broad; 1st segment 0.20 mm long, 0.18 mm broad, reddish black with 4 spines; 2nd segment 0.80 mm long, 0.14 mm broad with reddish black with 7 spines; 3rd segment 1.00 mm long, 0.20 mm broad, reddish black with 7 spines; 3rd segment 1.00 mm long, 0.20 mm broad, reddish black with 7 spines; claws 0.50 mm long, 0.18 mm broad, red.

ABDOMEN

28.00 mm long, 3.5 mm broad, bright yellowish, dorsum not tinged with bright brick-red, segment 1 to 4 pale yellow with black stripe dorsally; segment 5, 6, 7 and 8 yellowish with red transverse rings at basal region and black patches on dorsal side; segment 7, 8 and 9 with sharply defined black-mid-dorsal pyriform spots with narrow end of spots at base of segments. 10th segment with black quadrilateral spotl anal appendages reddish, changing to black towards apex; abdominal segments 8 and 9 parallel sided. Anal appendages (Figure 33): blackish with yellow base; superior 3.2 mm long, 0.38 mm broad with basally yellowish and apically blackish with dense black hairs laterally; inferior 1.40 mm long, 0.24 mm broad, reddish. Abdomen yellowish as entire breadth of hind wing.

COLOUR

Yellow: Abdomen, thorax, frons, anteclypeus, postclypeus, labium.

Blackish brown: Compound eyes.

Black: Mandible, ocelli, anal appendages.

PREY RECORD: Mosquitoes *Culex* sp., *Anopheles* sp., Moth *Sylepta derogata*.

HOLOTYPE: Male, India, Maharashtra, Coll. 2, 10-X-2004, Kusawade, Satara district M.S., Shinde K.P., antenna, leg on slide labelled as above, other parts with pined form, labelled as above.

PARATYPE: Male, Coll. 26-XII-2004 same data as above.

DISTRIBUTIONAL RECORD/OBSERVATIONS

Male 17, female 2. Ghanbi ♂2, 21-X-2004; Dicholi ♂1 9-I-2005; Tolewadi ♂1, 13-II-2005; Korgaon ♂1, 14-VIII-2005; Nechal ♂2 ♀1, 11-IX-2005; Dara ♂2, 9-X-2005; Rohine ♂3, 18-XII-2005; Patan ♂3♀1, 23-IV-2006; Zadoli ♂1 2-VII-2006; Yerad ♂1, 20-VIII-2006.

DISCUSSION

This species runs close to *Pantala flavescens* by having following characters:

1. Thorax dull yellowish.
2. Eyes reddish brown.
3. Discoidal cell.

However it differs from above species by having following characters:

1. Labrum brown.

2. Labium yellowish with brown border.
3. Hind wing and fore wing with bluish tinge and more transparent.
4. In hind wing apical line of discoidal cell with three nervures and not 2½ nervures.
5. Abdominal segment 8 and 9 parallel sided.
6. Fore wing antenodal nervures 16; postnodal nervures 8.
7. Hind wing antenodal nervures 8; postnodal nervures 10.
8. Flagellar formula: L/W; ½ = 8/4.87; $^{2/2}$ = 4.87/4.87; $^{3/2}$ = 29.41/4.87; $^{4/2}$ = 28.57/4.87; $^{5/2}$ = 33.3/4.87; A = 4.28.
9. Femora anterior half yellowish and posterior half blackish with 20 black spines.
10. Tarsus 1st segment longer than *Pantala flavescens*.
11. Trochanter whitish.
12. Abdomen is yellowish as entire breadth of hind wing.
13. Anal appendages blackish with yellow base.

PANTALA SHALAKHI SP.NOV.

MALE (Figures 34, 35)

49.00 mm in length excluding anal appendages; head 5.00 mm long; thorax 13.00 mm long, fore wing 45.00 mm long, hind wing 42.00 mm long, abdomen 31.00 mm long, yellowish with black, patches on dorsal side; superior anal appendages 3.60 mm long, black with dense hairs.

HEAD

5.00 mm long, 8.00 mm broad, roughly circular; occiput yellow, compound eyes reddish brown, occular space 4.00 mm, three ocelli in triangle, black with basally yellow ring, ocellar space 0.12 mm, interocelli space 2.00 mm; frons pale yellow with deep sulcus and dark yellow spots on front side; postclypeus pale yellow, anteclypeus pale yellow; labrum brownish; mandible black, mandible bases yellowish; labium brownish with middle lobe black.

Antenna

1.93 mm long, 0.20 mm broad, (width of scape 0.20 mm); scape 0.05 mm long, 0.20 mm broad; pedicel 0.30 mm long, 0.18 mm broad;

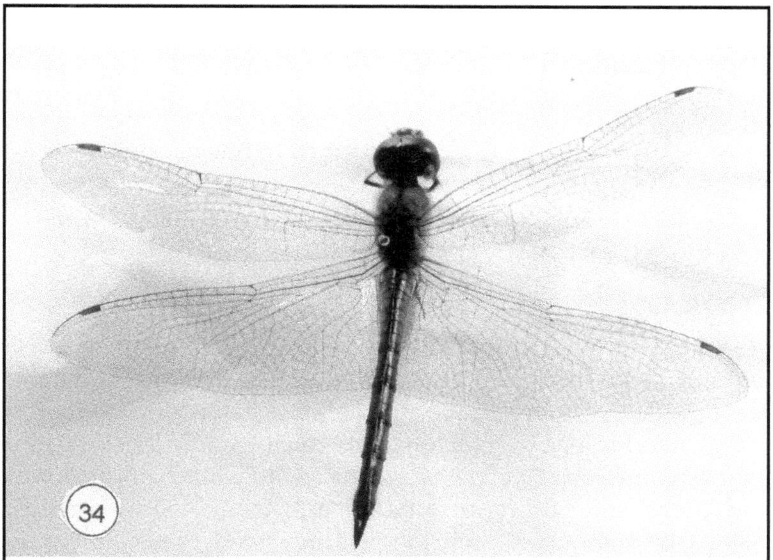

Figure 34: *Pantala shalakhi* sp.nov.; Male

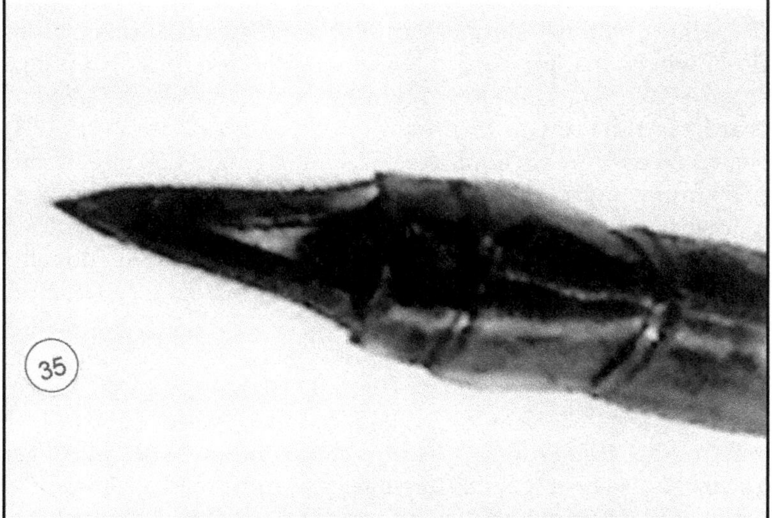

Figure 35: *Pantala shalakhi:* Anal Appendages; Male

flagellum: 5 segmented, 1.68 mm long, 0.041 mm broad; 1st segment 0.24 mm long, 0.041 mm broad; 2nd segment 0.32 mm long, 0.036 mm broad; 3rd segment 0.22 mm long, 0.019 mm broad; 4th segment 0.32 mm long, 0.010 mm broad; 5th segment 0.48 mm long, 0.009 mm broad.

Flagellar Formula

L/W; ½ = 5.85/8.88; $^{2/2}$ 8.88/8.88; $^{3/2}$ = 11.57/8.88; $^{4/2}$ = 32/ 8.88; $^{5/2}$ = 53/8.88; A = 2.50.

THORAX

13.00 mm long, 6.50 mm broad; yellowish greenish with dense white hairs on dorsolaterally; prothorax 7.00 mm long, 6.50 mm broad, yellowish greenish with dense white hairs dorsolaterally; 3 lobed, anterior lobe 0.7 mm long, brownish; middle lobe 6.00 mm long, 6.50 mm broad, yellowish greenish with white hairs on dorsal and lateral side; posterior lobe 0.3 mm long, 6.50 mm broad, yellowish; synthorax 6.00 mm long, 6.5 mm broad, robust, yellowish greenish no stripes on lateral side.

WINGS (Figure 34)

Wings hyaline; wing apices black and pointed; reticulation close, wing venation black; fore wing 45.00 mm long, 10.00 mm broad, 93.00 mm wing span; pterostigma 2.50 mm long, 0.76 mm broad, reddish brown with brown border; antenodal nervures 13½, postnodal nervures 8; hind wing 42.00 mm long, 14.00 mm broad, 87.00 mm wing span; pterostigma 2.00 mm long, 0.66 mm broad, reddish brown with black border; antenodal nervures 9, postnodal nervures 8; mahogany wings with yellowish brown veins and with yellowish tinge to both wings, apical line of discoidal cell in hind wing with 2¼ nervures.

LEG

Hind leg 15.06 mm long, 1.04 mm broad (width of coxa 1.04 mm); coxa 1.20 mm long, 1.04 mm broad, yellow with red tinge; trochanter 2 segmented, 1.80 mm long, 0.48 mm broad, yellowish; 1st segment 0.60 mm long, 0.40 mm broad; 2nd segment 1.20 mm long, 0.40 mm broad, 0.70 mm part of trochanter overlaps on femora; femora 4.14 mm long, 0.46 mm broad, yellowish on anterior side and posterior side black with 21 black pointed thick spine on inner side, last spine is longest, in 0.36 mm length; tibia 5.70 mm long, 0.28 mm broad, black with 21 black spines on inner side, spine 0.54 mm in length; outer side few yellow thin spines; tarsus 3 segmented, 1.96 mm in length and 0.18 mm broad; 1st segment 0.36 mm long, 0.16 mm broad with 4 spines on inner side; 2nd segment 0.60 mm long, 0.14 mm broad with 5 spines on inner side; 3rd segment 1.00 mm long, 0.18 mm broad with 18 spines on inner side, last spine is thickest than others, spine length 0.30 mm; claws red, 0.80 mm long, 0.20 mm broad with 4 red spines with black tip.

ABDOMEN

31.00 mm long, 4.00 mm broad, yellowish as half the length of hind wing with black patches; anterior segments broad and tapering posteriorly; segment 1st broad, yellowish with black spot on anterior side; segments 2nd and 3rd yellowish; segments 4, 5, 6, 7 and 8 yellowish with brown patches on lateral side, 10th segment parallel sided and with small black patch dorsally, 9th segment not parallel sided, bulging apically, narrow basally, 7, 8, 9 and other segments parallel sided; segments 9 and 10 brownish; Anal appendages (Figure 35): black with yellow base, 3.60 mm long, 0.50 mm broad; superior anal appendages 3.60 mm long, 0.40 mm broad with basally yellowish and apically dark black with dense black hairs on lateral side; inferior anal appendages 1.20 mm long, 0.50 mm broad, reddish.

COLOUR

Yellow: Occiput, coxa

Yellowish: Abdomen, frons, trochanter, thorax, postclypeus, anteclypeus.

Black: Anal appendages; ocelli, mandible.

Reddish brown: Compound eyes.

PREY RECORD: Moths, mosquitoes, jassids.

HOLOTYPE: Male, India, Maharashtra, Coll., 26-IX-2004; Kadoli, Satara district, M.S., Shinde, K.P., antenna, leg on slide labelled as above, other parts with pined form, labelled as above.

PARATYPE: Male 1, Coll. 20-IV-2005; same data as above.

DISTRIBUTIONAL RECORD/OBSERVATIONS

Male 13, female 1. Jungti ♂1 3-X-2004; Morgiri ♂1, 17-X-2004; Maldeo ♂1 19-XII-2004; Ghatmatha ♂1, 9-I-2005; Ghanbi ♂1 20-II-2005; Patan ♂3♀1 15-V-2005; Kusawade ♂2, 22-V-2005; Bamnoli ♂1, 5-V-2005; Yerad ♂2, 12-II-2006.

DISCUSSION

This species runs close to *Pantala flavescens* by having following characters:

1. Thorax dull yellowish.
2. Abdomen yellowish.
3. Discoidal cell.
4. Pterostigma reddish brown and similar in hind wing and fore wing.

However, it differs from above species by having following characters:

1. Labrum brownish.
2. Labium brownish.
3. Femora black entirely with big yellow stripe with 21 black spines.
4. Fore wing antenodal nervures 13½, post nodal nervures 8.
5. Hind wing antenodal nervures 9, post nodal nervures 8.
6. Flagellar formula: L/W; ½ = 5.85/8.88; $^{2/2}$8.88/8.88; $^{3/2}$ = 11.57/8.88; $^{4/2}$ = 32/8.88; $^{5/2}$ = 53/8.88; A = 2.50.
7. Abdomen yellowish as half the length of hind wing.
8. 10th segment parallel sided with small black patch dorsally. 9th segment not parallel sided bulging apically.
9. Anal appendages black with yellow base, narrow basally 3.60 mm long.
10. In hind wing apical line of discoidal cell with 2¼ nervures.

GENUS *ONYCHOTHEMIS* BRAUER

This genus is erected by Brauer in 1868. This genus is distributed in India, Sri Lanka, Myanmar, Malaysia, China, Java, Sumatra,

Borneo and the Philippines. Two species of this genus have been reported from India.

This genus is characterised by following features:

1. Head comparatively small.
2. Eyes contiguous for but a short distance.
3. Frons narrow, rather prominent.
4. Prothorax with moderately large posterior lobe, minutely emarginate and fringed with long hairs.
5. Thorax very robust.
6. Legs very long and robust.
7. Hind femora with 5 to 8 very robust, widely spaced spines.
8. Wings long and moderately broad, with close reticulation; discoidal cell in fore wing with short costal side, less than half the length of basal traverced.
9. Abdomen robust, broad, dorsoventrally at base and some what widened than tapering gradually to anal end and with a high middorsal keel or carina.

Onychothemis Brauer, Verh. Zool. bot. Ges. Wien, vol. xviii, pp. 170, 365, 732 (1868); Kirby, Trans. Zool. Soc. Lond. vol. xii, pp. 258, 284 (1889); id. id, Cat. Odon. p. 24 (1890); Karsch, Berlin Ent. Zeit. vol. xxxiii, p. 357 (1890); Kirby, Ann. Mag. Nat. Hist. (7) vol. xv, p. 277 (1905); Ris Cat. Selys, Fascs. ix, xiv. pp. 33, 833, 831 (1909, 1912); Fraser, J. Bombay Nat. Hist. Soc. vol. xxvi, pp. 742, 743 (1919).

ONYCHOTHEMIS PATANI SP.NOV.

MALE (Figures 36, 37)

43.00 mm body length excluding anal appendages; head 3.00 mm long; thorax 10.00 mm long; fore wing 31.00 mm long; hind wing 29.00 mm long; abdomen 29.00 mm long, yellow; superior anal appendages 0.8 mm long, black, hairy.

HEAD

4.00 mm long, 5.00 mm broad, moderately large, roughly triangular in front view; occiput yellow; Eyes widely contiguous, red, posteriorly yellow, occular space 3.00 mm; three ocelli in triangle, ocellar space 0.22 mm (diameter); interocellar space 0.36 mm, blackish

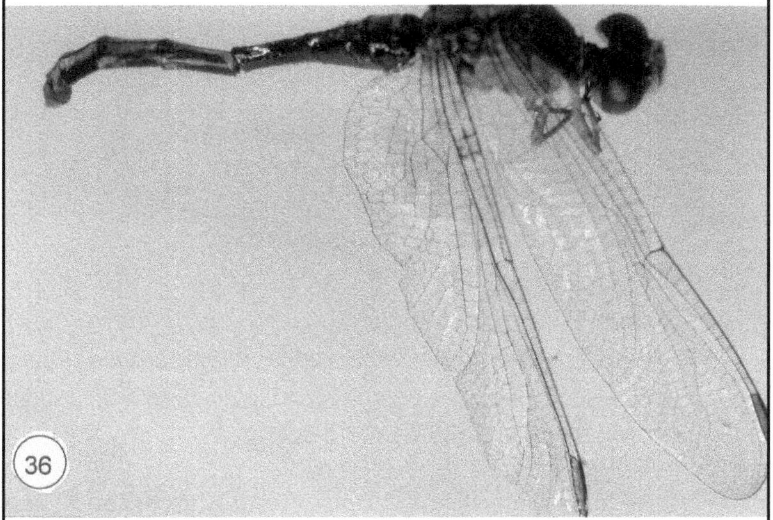

Figure 36: *Onychothemis patani* sp.nov.; Male

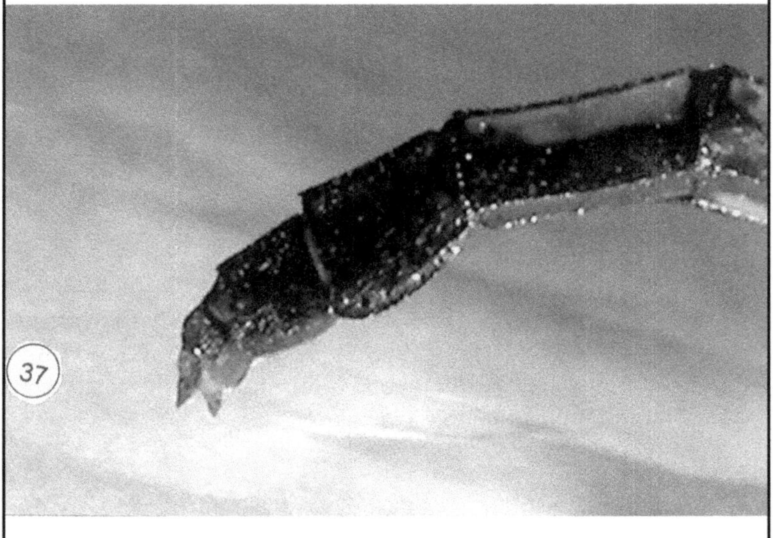

Figure 37: *Onychothemis patani:* Anal Appendages; Male

brown with red spot; frons dark yellow upper part, front pale yellow; postclypeus pale yellow, anteclypeus pale yellow, labrum dark yellow with two brown spots at mid region; mandible bases pale yellow; mandible brown; labium entire dark yellow.

Antenna

1.50 mm long; 1.6 mm broad, 7 segmented, brown with yellow rings, interantennal space 1.00 mm; scape 0.1 mm long, 0.16 mm broad; pedicel 0.22 mm long, 0.14 mm broad; Flagellum: 1.18 mm long, 0.04 mm broad; 1st segment 0.30 mm long, 0.04 mm broad; 2nd segment 0.20 mm long, 0.03 mm broad; 3rd segment 0.24 mm broad; 4th segment 0.20 mm long; 0.01 mm broad; 5th segment 0.24 mm long, 0.01 mm broad.

Flagellar Formula

(L/W) = ½ = 7.5/6.66; $^{2/2}$ = 6.66/6.66; $^{3/2}$ = 12/6.66; $^{4/2}$ = 20/ 6.66; $^{5/2}$ = 24/6.66; A = 2.1

THORAX

10.00 mm long, 4.00 mm broad; ground colour coppery brown, robust, hairy spiny; thorax coppery from laterally and ventrally; prothorax 5.00 mm long, 4.00 mm broad; anterior lobe 0.7 mm long, 4.00 mm broad, yellow, hairy with transverse plate; mid lobe, pale yellow, mid dorsally, red line, two yellow plates with black serrate border, Y shaped mark on mid dorsal, dorsally long, white hairs and short black many spines scattered, two brown broad lines on either sides, dorsally, laterally one yellow with two black spots; posterior lobe 0.3 mm long; 4.00 mm broad, yellow robust, 3 large plates yellow and one small dark yellow plate dorsally and one dorsal pale yellow laterally.

WINGS

Wing apices bordered by dark brown, not border by yellow; Fore wing 31.00 mm long, 7.00 mm broad; 66.00 mm wing span; transparent, hyaline; reticulation closed, black venation; antenodal nervures 13½; postnodal nervures 11; pterostigma 3.4 mm long, 0.46 mm broad, wing apices bordered with dark brown; Hind wing 28.00 mm long, 9.00 mm broad, 65.00 mm wing span; antenodal nervures 11; postnodal nervures 11, Cuii in hind wing arising from the posterior angle of discoidal cell; pterostigma 3.9 mm long, 0.70 mm broad. Hind wing apices pointed.

LEG

14.48 mm long, 1.10 mm broad; bluish yellow or grayish yellow at base; coxa, trochanter yellow, tibia black; coxa 1.30 mm long, 1.10 mm broad, outer small scanty yellow hairs, basal part of coxa overlaps on 1st segment of trochanter; trochanter 2 segmented, 1st segment 0.42 mm long, 0.50 mm broad, slightly triangular, yellow, 4 small yellow pointed spines and 4 small yellow hairs; 2nd segment 1.46 mm long, 0.60 mm broad; 0.80 mm part overlaps on femora, yellow, no hairs and spines, one big pale greenish or pale bluish patch; femora 4.24 mm long, 0.54 mm broad, outer side yellow, inner side black, outer side with row of small yellow spines at surface level, two black small, thick, pointed spines, 0.06 mm long at the junction of tibia and femora, two black spots, inner side with double row of small thick black, blunt spines, one big spine at basal region, 0.42 mm long, reddish tinge and one deep suture at basal region; tibia 4.46 mm long, 0.30 mm broad, black, with outer side, yellow strip with small, black blunt spines, at inner long black, thick pointed spines, apical and basal slightly smaller than middle, middle spine 0.60 mm long, 12 in number; tarsus 3 segmented, 1st segment 0.70 mm long, 0.16 mm broad with 3 spines and 3 hairs; 2nd segment 0.80 mm long, 0.18 mm broad with 6 spines and 7 hairs; 8th segment 1.10 mm long and 0.20 mm broad with 6 pairs of black spines. Claw 0.82 mm long, 0.20 mm broad with 2 spines, 0.50 mm long, brown, pointed.

ABDOMEN

29.00 mm long, 3.00 mm broad, cylindrical, anterior segments broad, 2.00 mm diameter and tapering middle then broad at posterior, segments, yellow; 1st segment yellow with two black patches and one yellow anule, 2nd segment yellow, 2 black annule transversly from 3rd to last segment, black mid dorsal spiny plate; segment 3rd with red patch; segments 4, 5, 6, 7 yellow; segment 8 yellow dorsally black, laterally; segments 9 and 10 complete black, two yellow spots on 9th segment, one yellow annule on 10th segment; superior anal appendages 2.92 mm long, 0.42 mm wide, yellowish brown at base, black at tip with hairs. Anal appendages (Figure 37): inferior anal appendages 1.60 mm long, 1.20 mm broad, triangular, yellow hairy.

COLOUR

Yellow: Abdomen, occiput, anteclypeus, postclypeus, labrum, labium, coxa, Trochanter, inferior anal appendages.

Brown: Mandible, antenna, inferior anal appendages, femora, tibia, tarsus, claws.

Ground coppery brown: Thorax.

HOLOTYPE: Male, India, Maharashtra, Coll., 4-IX-2005; Dara, Satara district, M.S., Shinde, K.P., antenna, leg on slide, labelled as above, other parts with pined form, labelled as above.

PARATYPE: Male 1, Coll. 6-XI-2006, same data as above.

DISTRIBUTIONAL RECORD/OBSERVATIONS

Male 14, Female 1. Bamnoli ♂2, 14-XI-2004; Patan ♂ 4, 19-XII-2004; Ghanbi ♂2, 1-I-2005; Kusawade ♂4, ♀1, 13-III-2005; Tapola ♂2, 6-III-2006.

DISCUSSION

This species runs close to *Onychothemis culminicola culminicola* Forster in Fraser's (1933) key by having following characters -

1. Short wings
2. Thorax coppery brown and
3. Pterostigma short.

However, it differs from above species by having following characters.

1. Labium and labrum dark yellow.
2. Legs bluish yellowish or greyish yellow at base.
3. Tibial and femoral spines, their number and structure.
4. Fore wing antenodal nervures 13½ and post nodal nervures 11.
5. Flagellar formula: L/W; ½ = 7.5/6.66; $^{2/2}$ = 6.66/6.66; $^{3/2}$ = 12/6.66; $^{4/2}$ = 20/6.66; $^{5/2}$ = 24/6.66; A = 2.1.
6. Anal appendages yellowish brown at base and inferior yellow with long grayish hairs.

GENUS *POTAMARCHA* KARSCH

The Genus *Potamarcha* was erected by Karsch in 1890. It is very similar to the genus *Cratilla*. The genus is moderate sized, never metallic coloured, blackish-brown, marked with yellow, but the markings often partly or entirely obscured by an overlay of bluish pruinescence. Head moderately large, eyes widely contiguous, thorax robust, abdomen parallel-sided, rather slim, cylindrical; genitalia of male small and inconspicuous, lamina hood shaped, depressed; hamules very similar to those of *Cartilla;* Genitalia of female small, vulvar scales hardly perceptible; wings long and narrow, reticulation close, node nearer pterostigma than base of wing.

Genotype, *Libellula obscura* Rambur.

Potamarcha Karsch, Berlin Ent. Zeit.Vol. xxxiii, p.370 (1800); Kirby. Cat. odon. p. 180 (1890); Ris, Cat. Call. Selys, Fasc. ix, pp. 21, 155, 156 (1909); Fraser, J. Bombay Nat.; Hist. Soc. Vol. xxv, p. 614 (1918); id; ibid. vol. xxvi, pp. 144, 145 (1918).

From India Fraser (1933) has described the only species, *Potamarcha obscura* (Rambur).

POTAMARCHA KOYNII SP.NOV.

MALE (Figures 38, 39)

43.00 mm in body length excluding anal appendages, head 3.00 mm long, thorax 12.00 mm long, fore wing 35.00 mm long, hind wing 36.00 mm long; abdomen 27.00 mm long, reddish brown, anal appendages 1.66 mm long, yellow.

HEAD

4.00 mm long, 4.00 mm broad, moderately large, roughly triangular in front view; occiput black; eyes widely contiguous reddish brown with black patches, occular space 2.00 mm; three occelli in triangle, ocellar space 0.3 mm (diameter); interocellar space 1.00 mm, blackish brown, at base yellow ring; frons yellowish brown and with deep sulcus, anteclypeus small yellow; postclypeus broad, brown; Labrum yellowish; mandible black; labium mid lobe brownish; convex anteriorly, lateral lobe not bordered or not black.

Antenna

Antenna 7 segmented, 2.44 mm long, 0.16 mm broad, filiform, blackish brown with yellow rings; scape 0.08 mm long, 0.18 mm broad; pedicel 0.3 mm long, 0.16 mm broad, brown, at tip yellow ring; 1st segment 0.4 mm long, 0.06 mm broad; 2nd segment 0.22 mm long, 0.09 mm broad; 3rd segment 0.26 mm long, 0.04 mm broad; 4th

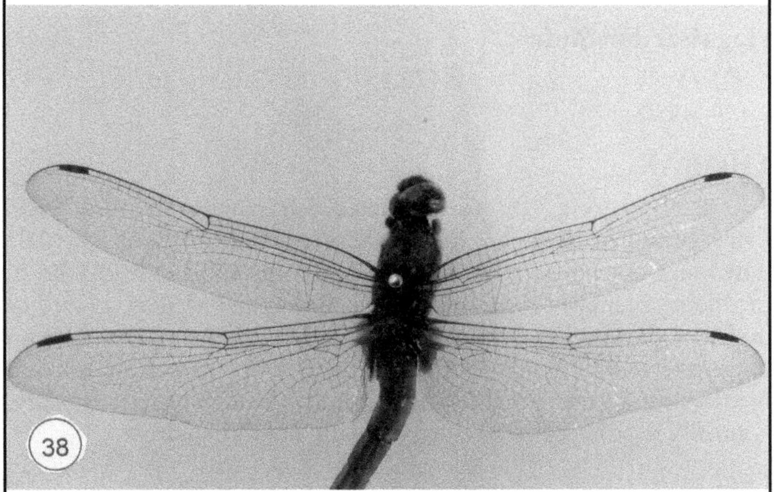

Figure 38: *Potamarcha koynii* sp.nov.; Male

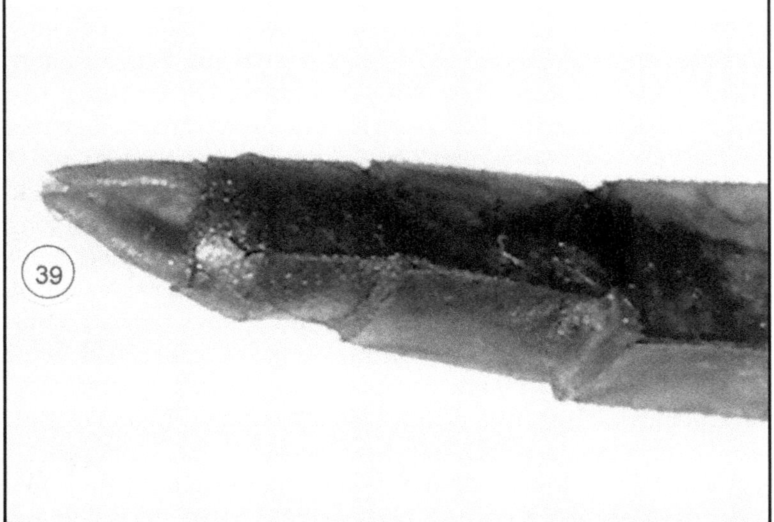

Figure 39: *Potamarcha koynii:* Anal Appendages; Male

segment 0.3 mm long, 0.03 mm broad; 5th segment 0.16 mm long, 0.02 mm broad.

Flagellar Formula

L/W ½ = 6.6/2.4; $^{2/2}$ = 2.4/2.4; $^{3/2}$ = 6.5/2.4; $^{4/2}$= 10/2.4; $^{5/2}$ = 8/ 2.4; A = 2.78.

THORAX

12.00 mm long, 5.00 mm broad, reddish brown with bluish tinge, hairy; prothorax 6.00 mm long, 5.00 mm broad; anterior lobe 0.02 mm long, not hairy, no transverse strip on middle; mid lobe of prothorax blackish, 5.00 mm long no transverse stripes on mid of middle lobe, laterally broken transverse line; posterior lobe 0.8 mm long; posterior lobe of prothorax small with no yellow border. Synthorax 6.00 mm long, 6.00 mm broad, blackish brown dorsally, ventrally reddish brown with externally not bluish tinge.

LEG

Hind leg 20.22 mm long, 1.3 mm broad, spiny, black and reddish brown toward base of femora; coxa 2.00 mm long, 1.2 mm broad, yellow with red and black patches; hairy at lateral side; Trochanter two segmented, 2.2 mm long; 1st segment 0.8 mm long, 0.56 mm broad, yellowish brown, few hairs; 2nd segment 1.94 mm long, 1.14 mm broad, leaf like part overlaps on femora, 0.6 mm broad, no spines, reddish brown; femora 5.6 mm long, 0.8 mm broad, outer side reddish brown, inner side black with 28 spines, spine 0.3 mm long, black, thick, blunt; outer side with scanty long hairs, hair 0.86 mm long black; tibia 5.5 mm long, 0.38 mm broad, black, 14 long spines inner side, spines 0.64 mm long; thick, black, pointed; outer side with 36 small spines, thick, black, blunt; basal part yellow; tarsus 3.5 mm long, 3 segmented; 1st segment 0.8 mm long, 0.22 mm broad, outer side reddish brown, inner side black with 4 spines, spines black, thick, pointed; 2nd segment 1.3 mm long, 0.24 mm broad, outer reddish brown, inner black, 5 black spines on inner side, thick, pointed; 3rd segment 1.4 mm long, 0.28 mm broad, outer side reddish brown with large black patch; on inner black 6 spines, spines thick, pointed, black; claws with 4 spines, 2 big, 0.9 mm long; 2 short 0.36 mm long, thick, brown with black tinge.

WINGS

Fore wing: 35.00 mm long, 8.00 mm broad, narrow, reticulation closed, transparent, well developed, wing span 74.00 mm; black well developed venation; pterostigma of fore wing slightly shorter in length than hind wing; posterior angle of discoidal cell of fore wing reaches to the half of the nervures of anal margin; pterostigma 2.64 mm long, 0.62 mm broad, yellowish brown, black, serrate margin (costal margin). Hind wing: span 75.00 mm, 36.00 mm long, 12.00 mm broad; pterostigma 2.70 mm long, 0.64 mm broad, yellowish brown with black margin, wing bases light yellow; posterior angle of hind wing discoidal cell is larger than *P. obsecura*.

ABDOMEN

27.00 mm long, 3.00 mm broad, parallel sided, rather slim cylindrical reddish brown, mid dorsally black patches; segments 8, 9, 10 are without yellow markings, 10th segment not black; Anal appendages (Figure 39) not black, broadly conical; superior anal appendages 1.66 mm long, 0.36 mm broad; inferior anal appendages 0.6 mm long, 0.22 mm broad, brownish with yellow inner side and scanty black hairs, lateral side with dense black hairs; dorsal side with few black hairs.

COLOUR

Reddish brown: Eyes, thorax, legs, abdomen.

Yellow: Anteclypeus, labrum, anal appendages

Yellowish brown: Frons, pterostigma.

Black: Occiput, mandible, wing venations.

Blackish brown: Antenna.

Brown: Postclypeus.

HOLOTYPE: Male, India, Maharashtra, Coll. 6-VI-2005; Kodoli, Satara district, M.S.; Shinde K.P.; antenna, leg on slide labelled as above, other parts with pined form, labelled as above.

PARATYPE: Male 1, Coll. 26-VI-2005; same data as above.

DISTRIBUTIONAL RECORD/OBSERVATIONS

Male 21, Female 2. Kodoli ♂ 5, ♀ 1, 26-IX-2004; Nechal ♂ 2, 5-XII-2004; Ghatmatha ♂ 2, 20-VI-2005; Urul ♂7, 4-XI-2005, Patan ♂4, ♀1, 28-V-2006; Yerad ♂2, 27-VIII-2006.

DISCUSSION

Potamarcha koynii sp.nov. runs close to *Potamarcha obscura* (Rambur) by having:

1. Labium yellow.
2. Occiput black.
3. Legs black.

However, it differs from above species by having following characters.

1. Frons yellowish brown
2. Labium mid lobe brownish, lateral lobes not bordered or not black.
3. No transverse stripes on mid of middle lobe of prothorax.
4. Flagellar formula: ½ = 6.6/2.4; $^{2/2}$ = 2.4/2.4; $^{3/2}$ = 6.5/2.4; $^{4/2}$ = 10/2.4; $^{5/2}$ = 8/2.4; A = 2.78.
5. Posterior angle of discoidal cell of fore wing reaches to the half of the nervures of anal margin.
6. Pterostigma of fore wing slightly shorter in length than hind wing.
7. Posterior angle of hind wing discoidal cell is larger than *P. obscura*.
8. Anal appendages not black and highly cone shaped, superior is with long tuft of hairs internally only tip is black.
9. Inferior anal appendages brownish.

PONTAMARCHA HUMANI SP.NOV.

MALE (Figures 40, 41)

40.00 mm long excluding anal appendages, head 4.00 mm long, thorax 11.00 mm long, abdomen 25.00 mm long, yellow with red patches, fore wing 30.00 mm long, hind wing, 31.00 mm long; superior anal appendages 1.00 mm long, yellow with yellow dense hairs on lateral side.

HEAD

4.00 mm long, 5.00 mm broad, roughly triangular, occiput yellow, compound eyes blackish brown, ocullar space 2.5 mm; three

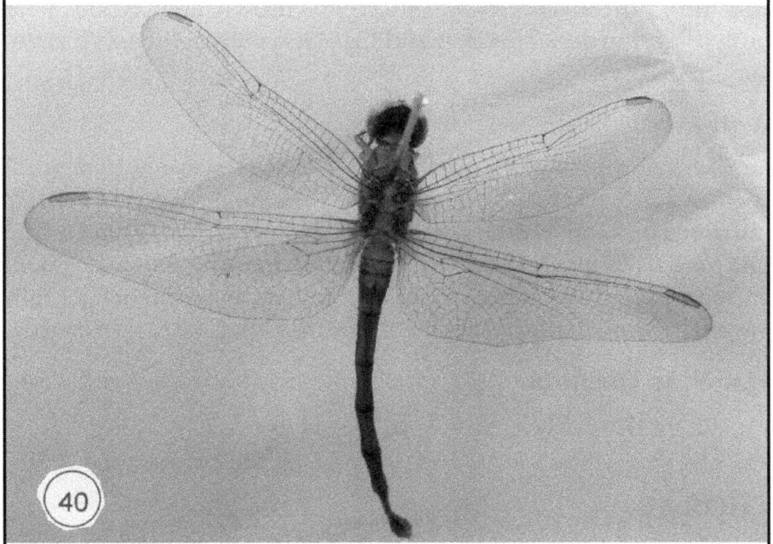

Figure 40: *Potamarcha humani* sp.nov.; Male

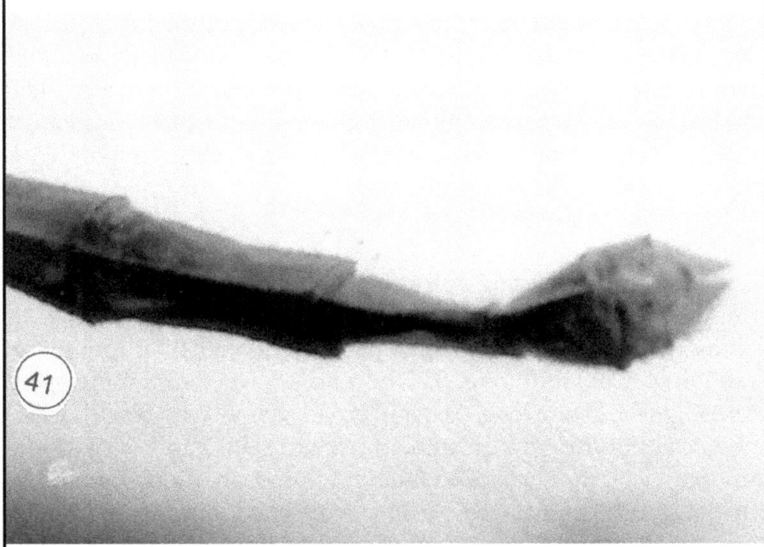

Figure 41: *Potamarcha humani:* Anal Appendages; Male

ocelli in triangle, black, ocellar space 0.18 mm interocellar space 1.50 mm; frons pale brown, postclypeus brown, anteclypeus pale brown, labrum dark brown, mandible black, mandible bases brown, labium yellow.

Antenna

1.84 mm long, 0.16 mm broad (width of scape 0.16 mm); 7 segmented, black; scape 0.06 mm long, 0.16 mm broad; pedicel 0.22 mm long, 0.14 mm broad. Flagellum: 5 segmented, 1st segment 0.32 mm long, 0.055 mm broad; 2nd segment 0.20 mm long, 0.04 mm broad; 3rd segment 0.24 mm long, 0.021 mm broad; 4th segment 0.24 mm long, 0.013 mm broad; 5th segment 0.56 mm long, 0.011 mm broad.

Flagellar Formula

L/W; ½ = 5.81/5; $^{2/2}$ = 5/5; $^{3/2}$ = 11.42/5; $^{4/2}$ = 18.46/5; $^{5/2}$ = 50.90/5; A = 3.66.

THORAX

11.00 mm long, 4.00 mm broad, yellow; prothorax 6.00 mm long, 4.00 mm broad yellow, with two black stripes laterodorsally with brownish black transverse stripe anteriorly; 3 lobed, anterior lobe 0.7 mm long, yellow with brown transverse stripe; mid lobe 5.00 mm long, 4.00 mm broad, yellow with middorsally side black spot and on dorsolaterally two black stripes; posterior lobe 0.3 mm long, 4.00 mm broad, yellow; synthorax 5.00 mm long, 4.00 mm broad, robust with dorsal side bright yellow and lateral sides yellow, a short black stripe on lateral side of mesothorax.

WINGS

Wings hyaline, wing apices black, pointed, reticulation close, wing venation black, wing bases rounded, both wing bases with yellow patches; hind pterostigma slightly longer than fore wing. Fore wing: 30.00 mm long, 8.00 mm broad, 63.00 mm wing span; pterostigma 3.20 mm long, 0.60 mm broad, yellow with black border; antenodal nervures 14, postnodal nervures 10. Hind wing: 31.00 mm long, 9.00 mm broad, 65.00 mm wing span; pterostigma 3.50 mm long, 0.70 mm broad, yellow with black border; antenodal nervures 11, post nodal nervures 11, discoidal cell with two nervures instead of three.

LEG

Hind leg: 14.84 mm long, 1.10 mm broad (width of coxa 1.10 mm); coxa 1.20 mm long, 1.10 mm broad, faint bluish with few black spots and one white spot; trochanter 2 segmented, 1.84 mm long, 0.56 mm broad, faint bluish; 1st segment 0.50 mm long, 0.50 mm broad, faint bluish with 3 brown small pointed curved spines on inner side; 2nd segment 1.34 mm long, 0.56 mm broad, 0.80 mm part overlaps on femora, faint bluish; femora 4.40 mm long, 0.60 mm broad, bright yellow with 11 brown pointed spines on inner side, last spine longest, last spine 0.48 mm long; on outer side 7 small pointed, brown spines at basal region; tibia 4.20 mm long, 0.28 mm broad, bright yellow outer side, red inner side, 11 spines on inner side, spine length 0.60 mm; 25 spines on outer side; tarsus 3 segmented, 2.60 mm long, 0.18 mm broad, red; 1st segment 0.70 mm long, red with 3 long spines, spine length 0.40 mm; 8 small pointed spines on outer side; 2nd segment 0.85 mm long, 0.16 mm broad, red with 4 spines, 3rd segment 1.90 mm long, 0.16 mm broad, red with 8 spines; red claws; 0.70 mm long, with black tip.

ABDOMEN

25.00 mm long, 2.5 mm broad, yellow and reddish brown, segment 1st yellow with one white transverse ring; segment 2nd yellow with 3 black transverse rings, segments 3, 4, 5, 6, 7, 8 and 9 reddish brown dorsally, black ventrally with each transverse black ring, segment 8th narrow at base and broad at anterior side, segment 10th reddish brown with big black patch on dorsal side; segment 10th yellow with two brown small spots on dorsal side, 10th segment shows feature of human face. Anal appendages (Figure 41): 1.00 mm long, 0.40 mm broad; superior anal appendages 1.00 mm long, 0.40 mm broad, yellow with dense yellow hairs, inferior anal appendages 0.40 mm long, 0.34 mm broad, yellow.

COLOUR

Yellow: Abdomen, anal appendages, occiput, labium, femora.

Faint bluish: Coxa, trochanter.

Brown: Labrum.

Blackish brown: Compound eyes.

Black: Mandible, antenna.

PREY RECORD: Mosquito *Culex* sp., jassid *Emoasca* sp. moths *Sylepta* sp.

HOLOTYPE: Male, India, Maharashtra, Coll. 21-XI-2004; Kadoli, Satara district, M.S., Shinde, K.P., antenna, leg on slide labelled as above, other parts with pined form, labelled as above.

PARATYPE: Male 1, Coll. 19-XII-2004 same data as above.

DISTRIBUTIONAL RECORD/OBSERVATIONS

Male 19, female 2. Patan ♂4, 26-XII-2004; Urul ♂5, 30-I-2005; Nisare ♂3, 19-VI-2005; Morgiri ♂1, 9-X-2005; Sondari ♂2, 20-XI-2005; Tapola ♂2♀1, 12-II-2006; Yerad ♂2 ♀ 9-IV-2006.

DISCUSSION

This species runs close to *Pontamarcha obscuta* (Rambur) by having following features:

1. Fore wing discoidal cell.
2. Labium yellow and
3. Occiput yellow.

However, it differs from above species by having following characters:

1. Labrum dark brown.
2. Thorax not dark brown.
3. By having black, transverse and dorsolateral stripes on prothorax.
4. Flagellar formula: L/W; ½ = 5.81/5; $^{2/2}$ = 5/5; $^{3/2}$ = 11.42/5; $^{4/2}$ = 18.46/5; $^{5/2}$ = 50.90/5; A = 3.66.
5. Hind discoidal cell with two nervures and not with three.
6. 10th abdominal segment shows feature of human face.
7. Anal appendage not black but yellow.
8. Legs not black but yellowish or faint bluish.

GENUS *INDOTHEMIS* RIS

The Genus *Indothemis* is raised by Ris in 1909. The genus is distributed in India, Sri Lanka, and Myanmar, Malaysia and Siam. It includes two species and one sub-species or geographical race.

The species of this genus resembles with the species of *Trithemis* but are easily distinguished by the borders of the discoidal field in the fore-wing diverging towards the wing-border, the opposite pertaining in *Trithemis*.

The genus is characterised by having following features

1. Moderate to small size, coloured black, in the adult or black marked with yellow in subadults.
2. Head moderately large; eyes broadly contiguous; frons with well-defined crest and shallow sulcus.
3. Prothorax with small posterior lobe; thorax robust;
4. legs slim, hind femora with about 12 evenly-sized robust spines and a longer one at distal end.
5. Abdomen slim and cylindrical, but slightly border at base and tapered very gradually to anal end.
6. Wings hyaline; reticulation close or moderately so; discoidal cell in fore wing with costal side angulated or not, short, much less than half the length of distal or basal sides, traversed or entire; that of hind wing entire, with base at level of arc; sectors of arc with a long fusion in fore and hind-wings; are situated between the first and second antenodal nervures; 8½ to 12½ antenodal nervures, the distal one incomplete; 1 cubital nervure in all wings; discoidal field beginning with 2 rows of cells, its borders diverging at wing-borders; no supplementing nervures to bridge; subtrigone in fore-wing 3 celled; pterostigma moderately long; mambrane very narrow. Genitalia of male small and inconspicuous in porfile, variable in the species; borders of segment 8 not dilated.

Indothemis Ris, Cat. Coll. Selys, Fasc. ix, p.29 (1909; id; ibid) Fraser, J. Bombay Nat. Hist. Soc. vol. xxvi, pp. 734, 735, Figure 43 (1919).

INDOTHEMIS INDICA SP.NOV.

MALE (Figures 42, 43)

53.00 mm body length excluding anal appendages; head 4.00 mm long; thorax 13.00 mm long; fore wing 34.00 mm long; hind wing 33.00 mm long; Abdomen 36.00 mm long, black with red patches

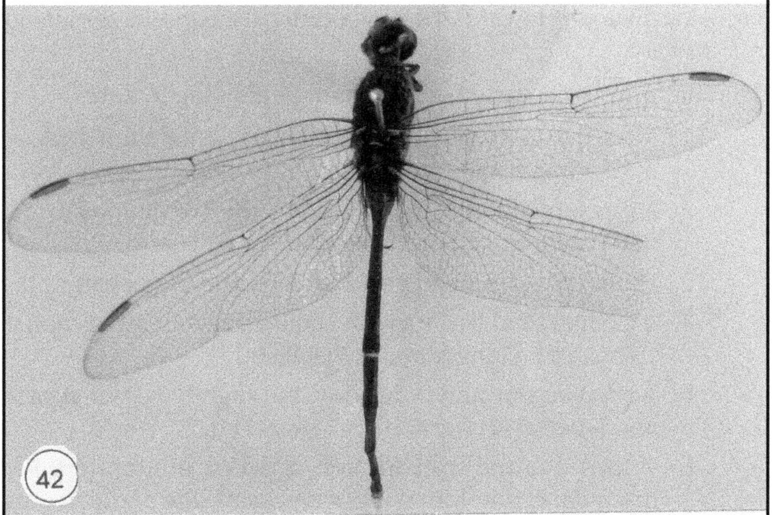

Figure 42: ***Indothemis indica*** **sp.nov.; Male**

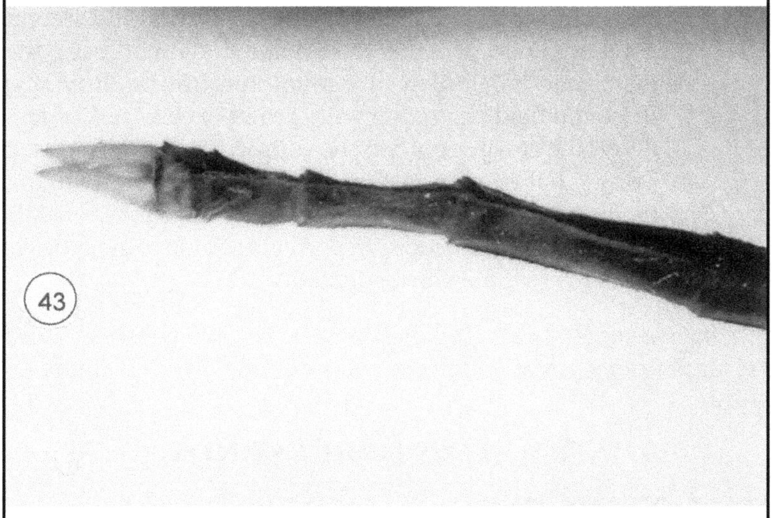

Figure 43: ***Indothemis indica:*** **Anal Appendages; Male**

dorsolaterally; superior anal appendages 1.8 mm long, yellowish, hairy.

HEAD

4.00 mm long, 6.00 mm broad, moderately large, roughly triangular in front view; occiput black with brown border; compound eyes widely contiguous, blackish brown with two yellow spots; occular space 3.00 mm; three occelli in triangle, ocellar space 0.3 mm (diameter); inter occllar space 0.42 mm, black, at base yellow ring; frons on an oblique plane, yellowish brown and with deep sulcus, at front one red spot with black border and one small black spot; anteclypeus small dull yellow; postclypeus broad dull yellow; Labrum yellowish brown with two small black spots; Labia mid lobe black, convex anteriorly, lateral lobe yellowish brown with dark brown spot at centre.

Antenna

7 segmented, 1.38 mm long, 0.16 mm broad, brownish with yellow rings; scape 0.08 mm long; Pedicel 0.3 mm long, 0.16 mm broad; 1st segment 0.3 mm long, 0.06 mm broad; 2nd segment 0.18 mm long, 0.09 mm broad; 3rd segment 0.2 mm long, 0.04 mm broad; 4th segment 0.2 mm long, 0.03 mm broad; 5th segment 0.2 mm long, 0.02 mm broad.

Flagellar Formula

L/W ½ = 5/2; $^{2/2}$ = 2/2; $^{3/2}$ = 5/2; $^{4/2}$ = 6/2; $^{5/2}$ = 10/2; A = 2.80.

THORAX

13.00 mm long, 5.00 mm broad, yellowish brown with black stripes, hairy; prothorax 7.00 mm long, 5.00 mm broad; anterior lobe 0.06 mm long, dense yellow hairy; middle lobe of prothorax 6.00 mm long, dorsally two yellowish brown stripes, dorsolaterally two reddish brown stripes, laterally one yellow and on either side two black stripes, dense yellow hairs; posterior lobe of prothorax 0.04 mm long, small reddish brown no border. Synthorax 6.00 mm long, 6.00 mm broad, reddish brown, tapering posteriorly, laterally two black small stripes, dorsally and laterally no hairs; ventrally dense hairs.

WINGS

Wings hyaline, apices very narrowly brownish for not more than 1 cell deep, bases of wings dark mahogany brown, restricted to bottom only, not reaching to distal of first antenodal nervure. Fore wing: 34.00 mm long, 8.00 mm broad, narrow reticulation closed, transparent, well developed, wing span 76.00 mm, pterostigma of fore wing 3.2 mm long, 0.76 mm broad, yellow with black border; Hind wing: span 69.00 mm, 33.00 mm long, 11.00 mm broad; pterostigma 3.00 mm long, 0.56 mm broad, yellow with black serrate border.

LEG

Hind leg 19.86 mm long, 1.4 mm broad, spiny, reddish brown and black towards tibia; coxa 0.5 mm long, 1.4 mm broad, reddish brown, faint black patch, scanty hairs; Trochanter two segmented, 1.80 mm long; 1st segment 0.8 mm long, 0.62 mm broad, reddish brown, 4 small black spines and few hairs; 2nd segment 1.72 mm long, 0.7 mm broad, leaf like 0.88 mm long flat plate covered femora; femora 6.22 mm long, 0.76 mm broad, reddish brown, 28 spines black, thick, pointed, longest 0.22 mm long, shortest 0.1 mm long; outer side with 29 hairs, hairs 0.42 mm long; tibia 6.12 mm long, 0.42 mm broad, inner side with 6 black, thick, pointed spines, spines 0.72 mm long, outer side of tibia with 38 small black, thick spines and few small hairs; tarsus three segmented, 3.82 mm long, 0.3 mm broad, black, spiny, 1st segment 1.04 mm long, 0.26 mm broad, 3 black, thick, pointed spines; 2nd segment 1.2 mm long, 0.2 mm broad, 6 black, thick, pointed spines; 3rd segment 1.58 mm long, 0.3 mm broad, 5 black, thick spines; claws with 4 spines, 2 big 1.2 mm long, 2 short spines 0.64 mm long, thick, pointed, brown, with black stripes, no black tip.

ABDOMEN

36.00 mm long, 3.00 mm broad, middle part slim, abdomen tappering posteriorly dorsally, first three segments broad, bulging, yellowish brown with black marking, rings on complete segment; segments 4,5,6 slender, slim, brown with black marking on end of the segment; segments 7,8,9 black, broad, laterally compressed, 10th segment 1.2 mm long, 1.5 mm broad, yellowish. Anal appendages (Figure 43): Superior anal appendages 1.8 mm long, 0.3 mm broad yellowish with black tip, with white dense hairs. Inferior anal appendages 0.5 mm long, white with black tip, with dense white hairs.

COLOUR

Black: Ocelli, labium mide lobe, coxa, tibia, spines, tarsus; 7,8,9 abdominal segments.

Blackish brown: Compound eyes.

Brown: Antenna.

Reddish brown: Synthorax, coxa trochanter, femora.

Yellow: Occiput, anteclypeus, postclypeus, pterostigma.

Yellowish: 10th abdominal segment, superior and inferior anal appendages.

HOLOTYPE: Male, India, Maharashtra, Coll. 3-VI-2005; Kodoli, Satara District, M.S.; Shinde K.P.; antenna, leg on slide labelled as above, other parts with pined form, labelled as above.

PARATYPE: Male 2, Coll. 17-VII-2005 same data as above.

DISTRIBUTIONAL RECORD/OBSERVATIONS

Male 14, Female 1. Kodoli ♂ 2, 3-X-2004; Nechal ♂1, ♀1, 5-XII-2004; Ghanbi ♂7, 17-XI-2004; Morgiri ♂2, 17-VII-2005.

DISCUSSION

This species run close to *Indothemis limbata limbata* (Selys) by following characters

1. Wings hyaline, apices very narrowly blackish brown for not more than one cell deep.
2. Bases of wings dark mahogany brown in hind wing.
3. Occiput black with brown border.

However, it differs from above species by following characters -

1. Legs not entirely black.
2. Femora reddish brown with 28 black spines.
3. Fore wing base not mahogany red.
4. Flagellar formula: L/W; ½ = 5/2; $^{2/2}$ = 2/2; $^{3/2}$ = 5/2; $^{4/2}$ = 6/2; $^{5/2}$ = 10/2; A = 2.80.
5. Thorax tapering posteriorly.

6. Pterostigma yellow with black border.
7. Abdomen considerably long, 36.00 mm.
8. Anal appendages yellowish, not black.
9. Posterior angle of discoidal cell of fore wing approaching anal margin, reaching outer marginal cell.

INDOTHEMIS KOYINEI SP.NOV.

MALE (Figures 44, 45, 46)

51.00 mm body length excluding anal appendages; Head 4.00 mm long; Thorax 12.00 mm long; Fore wing 37.00 mm long; Hind wing 35.00 mm long; Abdomen 35.00 mm long; brown with black patches; superior anal appendages 1.34 mm long, yellow.

HEAD

4.00 mm long, 6.00 mm broad, moderately large roughly triangular in front view, brown occiput yellow, hairy; Eyes widely contiguous blackish brown with 3 spots; occular space 3.00 mm; three ocell in triangle, inter ocellar space 0.44 mm; black at base yellow ring; frons on an oblique plane with deep sulcus, black yellow border; Anteclypeus narrow yellowish with small hairs; post and ant clypeus with small speresly scattered hairs, some light yellowish hairs on lateral side of post clypeus; postclypeus broad, yellow with brownish border anteriorly, 3 small hairs lateroposteriorly; Labrum yellowish, mandible yellow with brown teeth; Labium brown with two yellow spots on lateral lobe; middle lobe black anteriorly with small white hairs.

Antenna

7 segmented, 1.72 mm long, 0.22 mm broad, filiform, blackishbrown, scape 0.08 mm long; 0.22 mm broad, blackishbrown; pedicel 0.32 mm long, 0.14 mm broad blackishbrown; 1st segment 0.34 mm long, 0.06 mm broad; blackishbrown; 2nd segment 0.22 mm long, 0.04 mm broad; 3rd segment 0.28 mm long, 0.02 mm broad; 4th segment 0.20 mm long, 0.01 mm broad; 5th segment 0.28 mm long, 0.01 mm broad.

Flagellar Formula

L/W = ½ = 5.6/5.5; $^{2/2}$ = 5.5/5.5; $^{3/2}$ = 1.4/5.5; $^{4/2}$ = 20/5.5; $^{5/2}$ = 28/5.5; A = 2.62.

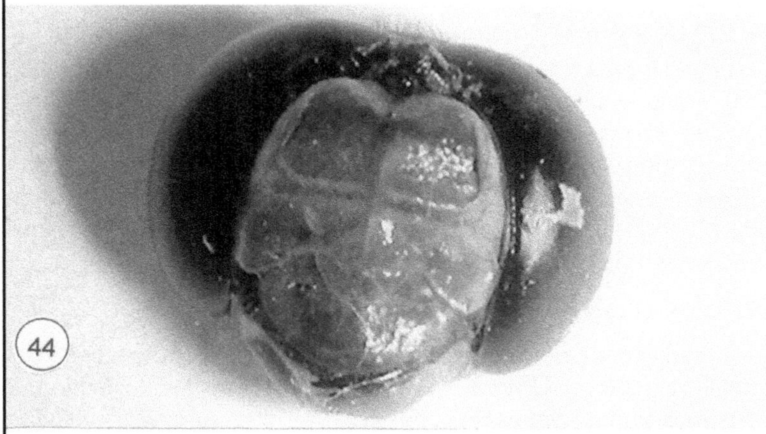

Figure 44: *Indothemis koyinei* sp.nov.; Male: Head

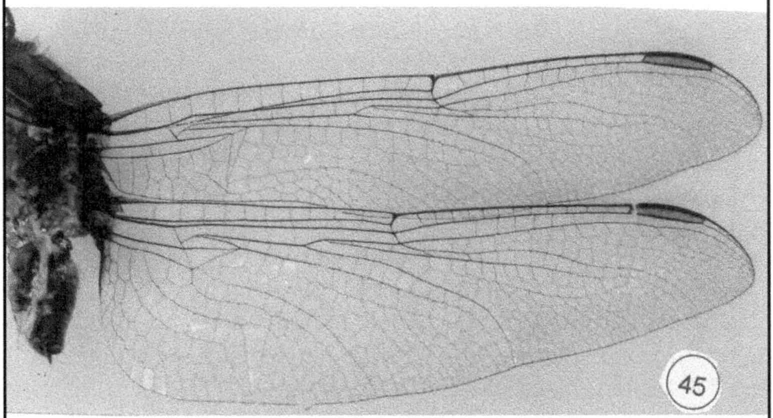

Figure 45: *Indothemis koyinei:* Male: Wings

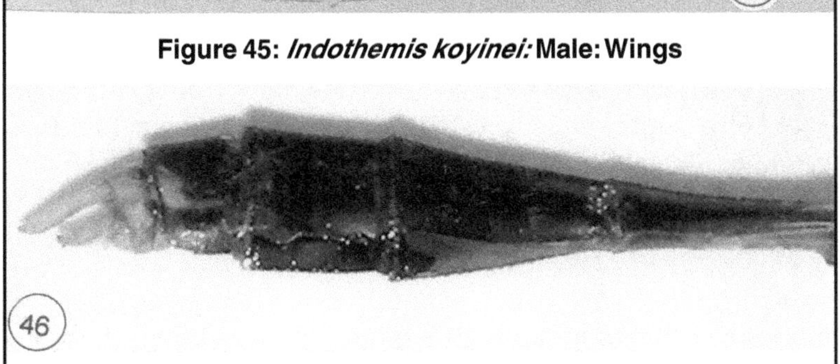

Figure 46: *Indothemis koyinei:* Anal Appendages; Male

THORAX

12.00 mm long, 4.00 mm broad, brown with blackish tinge; hairy; prothorax 6.00 mm long, 4.00 mm broad, 3 lobed anterior lobe 1.00 mm long, brown hairy, middle lobe of prothorax 4.5 mm long, blackish brown, dense hairy, one yellowish stripe and one black spot on mide dorsal; posterior lobe of prothorax 0.5 mm long, having yellow border; synthorax 6.00 mm long, 4.00 mm broad, brown, laterally one yellowish and two black stripes on border of pro and synthorax, one black stripe on metathorax.

WINGS (Figure 45)

Transparent, reticulation closed, well developed; fore wing 36.00 mm long, 8.00 mm broad, span 72.00 mm, black well developed venations, wings hyaline reticulation closed or moderately; fore wing anterior nodal nervures 15; posterior nodal nervures 10; pterostigma 3.3 mm long, 0.8 mm broad, yellow with black border; Hind wing span 67.00 mm, 35.00 mm long, 12.00 mm broad, round basal border; pterostigma 3.04 mm long, 0.7 mm broad, yellow with black border, basal yellow patch (mahogany); Hind wing anterior nodal nervures 13½ and postal nervures 10; apices of wing dark hyaline and narrowly bordered with blackish brown, base of hind wing with broad blackish brown marking.

LEG

Hind leg 21.10 mm long, 1.4 mm broad, reddish brown with black; coxa 2.00 mm long, 1.4 mm broad, reddish brown, fine yellow hairs; trochanter 2 segmented; 1st segment 0.8 mm, 0.66 mm broad, reddish brown, black patch, 2 small spines; 2nd segment 1.8 mm long, 0.72 mm broad, reddish brown, black patch, no spine and hair, 1.0 mm part overlap or covers femora; femora 6.00 mm long, 0.80 mm broad, black with large red patch, 5 white hairs, 0.36 mm long, 15 black spines, out of which one long at distal end, pointed, thin, 0.56 mm long, 18 small thin black spines 0.6 mm long. Tibia 5.76 mm long, 0.40 mm broad, black with red spots, 10 spines, black, thick, pointed, 0.80 mm long; tarsus 3 segmented, black; 1st segment 0.90 mm long, 0.22 mm broad, black with red tinge, 3 long spines, thick, pointed; 2nd segment 1.10 mm long, 0.20 mm broad, 3rd segment 1.54 mm long, 0.28 mm broad with 9 spines, black red tinge, 9 spines thick black pointed, 0.30 mm long; claw with 4 spines, red, black patch, 2 long spines, 1.20 mm long, 2 short spines, 0.56 mm long.

ABDOMEN

35.00 mm long, 3.00 mm broad, cylindrical tapering posteriorly; brown with black patches; mid dorsally black line; 1, 2, 3 segments compact broad, ventrally floopy, rounded, blackish brown 4, 5, 6, 7 segments yellow, longitudinal stripe on dorsal side of segments 4, 5, 6; Abdomen angulate between 6th and 7th, cylinder with yellow segment; 8,9, 10 and dorsolaterally compressed, 10th segment black with one yellow spot; segments 4 to end black marked with yellow, segments. 4 to 7 yellow with black rings. Superior anal appendages 1.34 mm long, 0.28 mm broad, hairy, yellow, inferior, anal appendages (Figure 46), 0.72 mm long, 0.26 mm broad, triangular, yellow, dense hairy; superior anal appendages knife like not hooked.

COLOUR

Yellow: Occiput, anal appendages, postclypeus, labrum.

Blackish brown: Compound eyes, antenna

Black: Ocelli, frons, anteclypeus, femora, tarsus

Brown: Thorax, abdomen.

Reddish brown: Coxa, trochanter.

HOLOTYPE: Male, India, Maharashtra, Coll. 19-XII-2004, Kusawade, Satara district, M.S.; Shinde, K.P.; Antenna, leg on slide labelled as above, other parts with pined form labelled as above.

PARATYPE: Male 1, Coll. 30-I-2005; same data as above.

DISTRIBUTIONAL RECORD/OBSERVATIONS

Male 11, Female 1. Kusawade ♂2, 19-XII-2004; Yerad ♂3 21-VII-2005; Bamnoli ♂1, ♀1, 4-IX-2005; Kadoli ♂1 20-XI-2005; Navaja ♂2, 22-I-2006; Dara ♂2, 7-V-20006.

DISCUSSION

This species runs close to *Indothemis limbata limbata* (Selys) by having following characters:

1. Apices of wings finely bordered with blackish brown, antenodal nervures 13½ in forewing.

However, it differs from the above species by having following features:

1. Abdomen length 85 mm long.
2. Labrum and labium yellowish black.
3. Posterior clypeus with lateral spines and full of light yellow hairs on lateral side of postclypeus.
4. Abdominal stripes.
5. Flagellar formula: (L/W); ½ = 5.6/5.5; $^{2/2}$ = 5.5/5.5; $^{3/2}$ = 14/5.5; $^{4/2}$ = 20/5.5; $^{5/2}$ = 28/5.5; A = 2.62.
6. Superior anal appendages yellow knife like, not hooked.

GENUS *NEUROTHEMIS* BRAUER

The genus *Neurothemis* is raised by Brauer in 1842. This genus is distributed in Tropical Asia, Sundale Archipelago, Borneo, New Guinia, Philippines and Australia. The genus consists of several closely related species. Seven species have been reported from India. Two of which are found in Sri Lanka. All breed in swamps, marshes or stagnant waters and are generally found in large colonies in the neighbourhood of their watery habitat.

This genus is characterised by following features:

1. Dragonflies of moderate size.
2. Wings are partly or wholly coloured in one or both sexes and often by a very close reticulation of the wings.
3. Body usually coloured some shade of yellow or reddish brown.
4. Head moderately large; eyes rather shortly contiguous; frons rounded, but with well-defined crest in the male, less so in the female; vesicle large, slightly notched.
5. Prothorax with small posterior lobe, arched and slightly emarginate; thorax robust.
6. Legs moderately long and slim, hind femora with a row of rather numerous, gradually lengthening spines.
7. Abdomen relatively short, slightly dilated dorsoventrally at base, then slim and tapered very gradually to the end; rather compressed and subcylindrical in the female.

8. Wings rather broad; reticulation close, a secondary closer reticulation often present in the coloured basal parts of wings; discoidal cell of fore wing rather broad, costal side half the length or more than half the length of distal and basal sides, transversed or filled with a close network of nervures; discoidal cells of hind wing with base at level of arc, traversed, often many times, distal side markedly concave; sectors of arc with short fusion in fore wing, a long fusion in the hind; arc lying between the first and second antenodal nervures; antenodal nervures never less than 11½, distal one complete in fore wing. Supplementary nervures to the bridge present; subtrigone in fore wing with 3 or numerous cells; pterostigma and membrane moderately large.

Genotype, *Libellula fulcia* Drury, *Polyneura* Rambur, Ins. Nevrop. p. 26 (1812); Hagen, Stett. Ent. Zeit. Vol. X, p. 170 (1849).

Neurothemis Brauer, Verh. Zool. bot. Ges. Wien, vol. xvii, pp. 6, 289 (1867); id., Ibid. vol. xviii, pp. 366, 717 (1868); Selys, Ann. Mus. Civ. Genova, vol. xiv, p. 290 (1874); Kirby, Trans, Zool. Soc., Lond. Vol. xii, pp. 260, 271 (1889); Forster, Termeszetr. Fase xxi, p. 273 (1898); Kruger, Stett. Ent. Zeit, vol. lxiv, p. 248 (1903); Ris, Cat. Coll. Selys, Fascs, ix and xiii, pp, 29, 548-553 (1909, 1911); Fraser J. Bombay Nat. Hist. Soc. Vol-xxvi, pp. 506-508 (1919).

NEUROTHEMIS TULLIA TULLIA DRURY (Figure 47)

Libellula tullia DRURY, III. Exot. Ins. Vol. ii, Pi, xivi, Figure 3, p. 85 (1773).

Libellula equestris Fabricius, spec. Ins. Vol. 1. P. 523 (1781); id., Ent. Syst. P.379 (1793); Burmeister, Handb, Ent. Vol. ii, p. 855 (1839); Rambur, Ins. Nevrop p. 79 (1842); Hagen, Stett. Ent. Zeit. Vol. X, p. 175 (1849); id., Verh., Zool. not., Ges, Wien, Vol. viii, p. 480 (1858); Calvert, Trans. Amer. Ent. Soc. Vol. xxv, p. 77 (1898).

Libellula lineata Fabricius, Ent. Syst. Vol. ii. p. 375 (1793); Rambur Ins. Nevrop. p. 73 (1842), *Diplax equestrix* Brauer, Novara, p. 104 (1866). *Neurothemis equestris* Brauer, Verh. Zool. bot. Ges. Wien. Vol., xviii, p. 718 (1868); Selys, Ann. Mus. Civ. Genova, vol. xiv, pp. 290, 297 (1879); id., Ibid, Vol. xxx, p. 447 (1891); Kruger, Stett., Ent, Zeit,

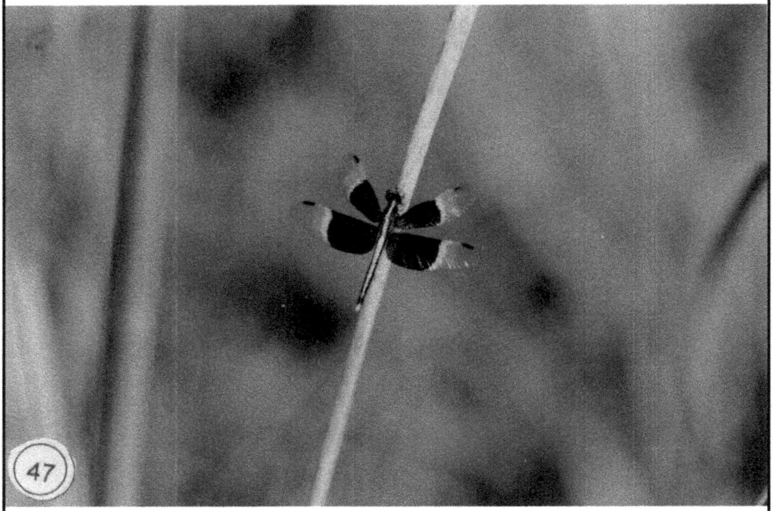

Figure 47: *Neurothemis tullia tullia*; Male

vol. Ixiv. P. 257 (1903); Martin, Mission pavie, Zool. p. 5 (Sep.) (1904). *Neurothemis tullia* Kirby, Cat, Odon. p. 8 (1890); id.; J. Linn. Soc., Zool. Vol. xxiv, p. 550 (1893); id., Ann., Mag, Nat. Hist, (6) Vol. xiv, p. 112 (1894); id., ibid. (7) vol. V.P. 531 (1900); Laidlaw, Proc. Zool. Soc. Lond. part I, p. 66 (1902); Kirby, Ann. Mag. Nat. Hist., (7) Vol. xv, p.271 (1905); Laidlaw, Rec. Ind. Mus. Vol. viii, p. 337 (1914); id., J. F.M.S. Mus, Vol. xvi, p. 225 (1930).

Neurothemis tullia Feralis Ris, Cat. Coll. Selys, Fase. xiii, pp. 551, 561, 562 (1911). Fraser, J. Bombay Nat. Hist. Soc. Vol. xxvi, pp. 507,510, 511 (1919); id., J. Nat. Hist. Soc. Siam Vol. iii, p. 458 (1919); id., Rec. Ind. Mus. Vol. xxvi, pp. 428, 437 (1924); id., J. Siam. Soc., Nat. Hist., Suppl. Vol. vii, p. 85 (1927); id., Rec. Ind. Mus. Vol. xxxiii p. 446 (1931).

MALE (Figure 47)

31.00 mm long excluding anal appendages; head 3.00 mm long; thorax 9.00 mm long; fore wing 25.00 mm long; hind wing 24.00 mm long; abdomen 19.00 mm long, black; anal appendages 1.1 mm long, creamy white tipped with black.

HEAD

3.00 mm long, 4.2 mm broad, roughly triangular, occiput black; compound eyes blackish brown above, violanceous below; occular space 2.1 mm; three ocelli in triangle, brown with yellow basal ring; ocellar space 0.21 mm; inter ocellar space 00.68 mm; frons black, postclypeus blackish; anteclypeus black; labrum black; labium blackish brown, middle lobe and border of lateral lobes paler brown.

ANTENNA

7 segmented antenna, blackish, 1.14 mm long, 0.11 mm broad (width of scape 0.11); scape 0.5 mm long, 0.11 mm broad; pedicel 0.19 mm long, 0.09 mm broad. Flagellum: 5 segmented, 0.90 mm long, 0.038 mm broad; 1st segment 0.21 mm long, 0.038 mm broad; 2nd segment 0.18 mm long, 0.031 mm broad; 3rd segment 0.21 mm long, 0.024 mm broad; 4th segment 0.14 mm long, 0.017 mm broad; 5th segment 0.16 mm long, 0.012 mm broad.

Flagellar Formula

L/W; ½ = 5.52/5.80; $^{2/2}$ = 5.80/5.80; $^{3/2}$ = 8.75/5.80; $^{4/2}$ = 8.23/5.80; $^{5/2}$ = 13/5.80; A = 1.42.

THORAX

9.00 mm long, 3.8 mm broad, black, mid-dorsal carnia of thorax narrowly yellow; prothorax 4.90 mm long, 3.8 mm broad, prothorax 3 lobed; anterior lobe 0.6 mm long, mid lobe 3.9 mm long, 3.8 mm broad, posterior lobe 0.4 mm long, 3.8 mm broad; synthorax 5.1 mm long, 3.8 mm broad, black.

WINGS

Wings hyaline for apical half, opaque, steely blue-black for basal half, the border of this opaque area running in both fore and hind wings from costal border, one cell distal to mid in fore wing, two or 3 cells distal in hind to the posterior border of wings in a convex curve; a broad opalescent white band bordering the black area in both wings, border at costal border, tapering to posterior border but not quite attaining to it; Fore wing: 25.00 mm long, 7.00 mm broad; wing span 53.00 mm; antenodal nervures 7, post nodal nervures 10½; pterostigma 2.7 mm long, 0.61 mm broad, brown; discoidal cell transversed twice in fore wing; Hind wing: 24.00 mm long, 8.00 broad, 51.00 mm wing span; pterostigma 2.6 mm long, 0.62 mm broad, brown; antenodal nervures 8, post nodal nervures 10; cubital nervures 5 present in fore wing, cubital nervures 2 in hind wing.

LEG

Hind leg 16.10 mm long, 1.10 mm broad (width of coxa 1.10 mm) black; tibia black exterior yellow; coxa 1.40 mm long 1.10 mm broad, yellow, trochanter 2 segmented, 1.84 mm long 0.41 mm broad; 1st segment 0.44 mm long, 0.41 mm broad, yellowish brown; 2nd segment 0.70 mm long, 0.54 mm broad, brown; femora 4.50 mm long, 0.58 mm broad, blackish brown; tibia 4.70 mm long, 0.32 mm broad, blackish, exterior yellow; tarsus 3 segmented, 3.56 mm long, 0.24 mm broad, black; claw 0.60 mm long, brown.

ABDOMEN

19.00 mm long, 2.3 mm broad; a broad mid dorsal interrupted creamy white stripe on segments, 1 to 8, broad at base of segments, tapering to apical end and becoming lost on segment 8, superior anal appendages 1.1 mm long, 0.5 mm broad, creamy-white tipped with black.

COLOUR

Black: Abdomen, occiput.

Creamy white: Superior anal appendages.

Blackish brown: Compound eyes.

Brown: Ocelli.

HOLOTYPE: Male, India, Maharashtra, Coll. 19-XII-2004; Nisare, Satara district, M.S. Shinde K.P., antenna, leg on slide, labelled as above, other parts with pinned form, labelled as above.

PARATYPE: Male 1, Coll. 20-IV-2005; same data as above.

DISTRIBUTIONAL RECORD/OBSERVATIONS

Male 9, Female 1. Patan ♂2, ♀1, 14-XI-2004; Navaja ♂1, 16-I-2005; Ghatmatha ♂1, 3-VII-2005; Kamargaon ♂2, ♀1, 18-XI-2005; Morgiri ♂2, 12-II-2006; Jungti ♂1, 5-III-2006.

GENUS *BRADINOPYGA* KIRBY

This genus *Bradinopyga* was erected by Kirby in 1893. It is distributed in Africa and peninsular India. From India only one species have been reported. However, the species is widely spread throughout the plain. Where it breed in small pools, wells etc. The genus is characterized by following features.

1. Dragonflies are moderate sized with cryptic colouring in black, grays and white, and with hyaline wings.
2. Head moderately large; eyes broadly contiguous.
3. Frons with crest rounded, sulcus narrow and deep; vesicle rounded or notched.
4. Prothorax with small, rounded, posterior lobe; thorax robust.
5. Legs rather short, slim; hind femora with numerous closely set short spines.
6. Abdomen slightly dilated at base, then very narrow, triquetral, dorsum strongly ridged.
7. Wings hyaline, long and moderately narrow, reticulation close or very close; discoidal cell in fore wing narrow, costal side less than half the length of basal and distal sides.
8. Pterostigma of moderate size, bicolorous; membrane large.

Genotype–*Libellula geminata*, Rambur.

Bradinopyga Kirby J. Linn. Soc. Zool. Vol. xxiv, p. 553 (1893); Calvert. Proc. Acad. Phil. p. 241 (1899); Ris. Cat. Coll. Selys, fascs. ix-xiii pp. 29. 544-555 (1910-1911); Fraser J. Bombay Nat. Hist. Soc. vol. xxvi, p. 514 (1919).

Apeleutherus Kirby, Ann. Mag. Nat. Hist. (7) Vol. vi p. 73 (1900).

BRADINOPYGA SATARENSIS SP.NOV.

MALE (Figure 48, 49)

Body 43.00 mm long excluding anal appendages; head 7.00 mm long, thorax 10.00 mm long, fore wing 35.5 mm long, hind wing 34.00 mm long, abdomen 26.00 mm long, black with yellow bands, anal appendages 1.72 mm long, yellow with hairs.

HEAD

7.00 mm long, 5.00 mm broad; occiput blackish brown; compound eyes brown, occular space 2.5 mm; three ocelli in triangle, brown with yellow ring, ocellar space 0.24 mm long, interocellar space 1.20 mm; frons dark black with deep sulcus; postclypeus dull

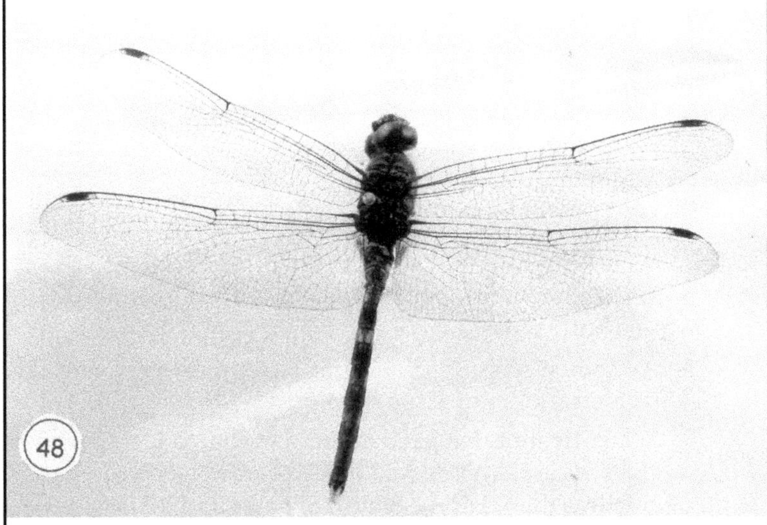

Figure 48: *Bradinopyga satarensis*; Male

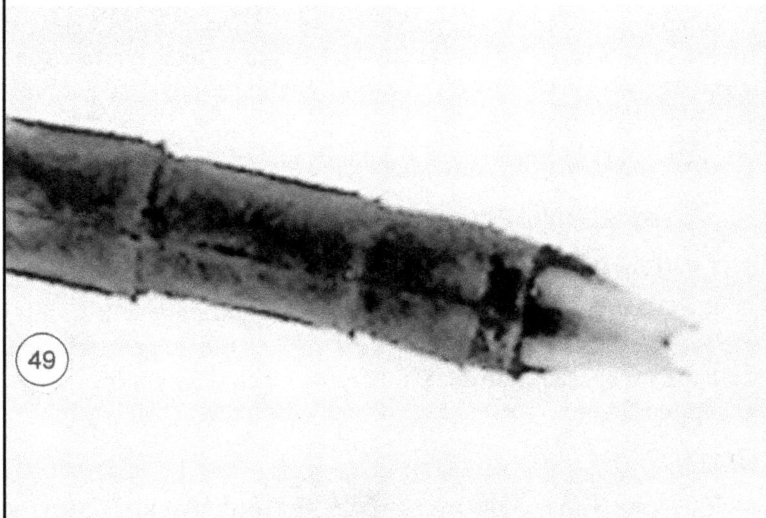

Figure 48: *Bradinopyga satarensis:* Anal Appendages; Male

yellowish, anteclypeus black, labrum brown; mandible black, mandible bases yellowish; labium dark yellow with black spots.

Antenna

2.10 mm long, 0.12 mm broad (width of scape 0.12 mm); 7 segmented, black; scape 0.04 mm long, 0.12 mm broad; pedicel 0.20 mm long, 0.10 mm broad. Flagellum: 5 segmented, 1.86 mm long, 0.04 mm broad; 1st segment 0.40 mm long, 0.04 mm broad; 2nd segment 0.24 mm long, 0.031 mm broad; 3rd segment 0.22 mm long, 0.023 mm broad; 4th segment 0.60 mm long, 0.016 mm broad; 5th segment 0.40 mm long, 0.010 mm broad.

Flagellar Formula

L/W; ½ = 10/7.74; $^{2/2}$ = 7.74/7.74; $^{3/2}$ = 9.56/7.74; $^{4/2}$ = 37.5/ 7.74; $^{5/2}$ = 40/7.74; A = 2.70.

THORAX

10.00 mm long, 5.5 mm broad, robust, blackish brown with dense hairs and yellow spots; prothorax 6.00 mm long, 5.5 mm broad, blackishbrown with dense hairs and yellow spots, 3 lobes; anterior lobe 0.6 mm long, blackish brown with hairs; middle lobe 4.6 mm long, 5.5 mm broad; blackish brown with hairs on dorsolateral side and 2 yellow spots on lateral side; posterior lobe 0.3 mm long, 5.5 mm broad, brown with hairs; synthorax 4.00 mm long, 5.5 mm broad, robust with black dorsally and blackishbrown laterally.

WINGS

Wings hyaline, wing apices broad and pointed; reticulation close, wing venation black, wing bases rounded. Fore wing: 35.5 mm long, 7.00 mm broad; wing span 74.00 mm; pterostigma 3.20 mm long, 0.80 mm broad, black centrally and both anterior and posterior sides yellow, pterostigma border black; antenodal nervures 12, postnodal nervures 9; supporting anterior and posterior cells marked with dark black border. Hind wing: 34.00 mm long, 10.5 mm broad, 71.00 mm wing span; pterostigma 3.00 mm long, 0.80 mm broad, black at centre and both anterior and posterior side yellow, pterostigma border black; antenodal nervures 9, postnodal nervures 8.

LEGS

Hind leg 12.73 mm long, 1.00 mm broad, coxa 0.80 mm long, 1.00 mm broad, yellow with dense yellow hairs; trochanter 2 segmented, 0.90 mm long, 0.50 mm broad, yellowish black; 1st segment 0.40 mm long, 0.50 mm broad, yellowish black; 2nd segment 0.50 mm long, 0.44 mm broad, yellowish black; femora 4.60 mm long, 0.46 mm broad, blackish with 4 spines; tibia 4.40 mm long, 0.26 mm broad with 9 black, thin, long, pointed spines, spine 0.50 mm long; tarsus 3 segmented, 1.32 mm long, 0.22 mm broad; black with spines; 1st segment 0.24 mm long, 0.22 mm broad with 2 spines; 2nd segment 0.60 mm long, 0.22 mm broad, black with 3 spines; 3rd segment 0.50 mm long, 0.20 mm broad, black with 3 spines; claw 0.70 mm long, 0.22 mm broad, black with 2 spines.

ABDOMEN

26.00 mm long, 3.00 mm broad, black with yellow stripes; 1st segment dorsally yellow and laterally black; 2nd segment black with yellow spot on dorsal side, segment 3 black; segments 4, 5, 6, 7 and 8 black with yellow transverse rings, segments 9 and 10 black; Anal appendages (Figure 49): 1.72 mm long, 0.60 mm broad, yellow with hairs; superior anal appendages cylindrical, 1.72 mm long, 0.42 mm broad, yellow with black tips and black hairs; inferior anal appendages 1.30 mm long, 0.60 mm broad, yellow with black tip.

COLOUR

Black: Abdomen, frons, mandible, antenna, tibia, tarsus, claws, femora.

Yellow: Anal appendages, coxa, trochanter.

Brown: Compound eyes, ocelli,

Blackish brown: Thorax.

PREY RECORD: Midges, *Contarinia* sp.

HOLOTYPE: Male, India, Maharashtra, Coll. 19-XII-2004; Rohine, Satara district, M.S., Shinde K.P., antenna, leg on slide labelled as above, other parts with pined form, labelled as above.

PARATYPE: Male 1, Coll. 2-X-2005, same data as above.

DISTRIBUTIONAL RECORD/OBSERVATIONS

Male 24, female 1. Patan ♂1, 12-IX-2004; Yerad ♂1♀1, 19-IX-2004; Dara ♂2, 7-XI-2004; Ghanbi ♂3, 26-XII-2004; Bamnoli ♂4, 13-II-2005; Ghatmatha ♂2, 27-II-2005; Tapola ♂2, 10-IV-2005; Kusawade ♂4, 8-V-2005; Munawale ♂3, 14-VIII-2005; Morgiri ♂1, 18-IX-2005; Navaja ♂1, 19-II-2006.

DISCUSSION

This species runs close to *Bradynopyga geminata* (Rambur) by following characters:

1. Abdomen black with yellow marking.
2. Pterostigma.
3. Discoidal cells in wings.

However, it differs from the above species by having following features:

1. Labrum brown.
2. Labium dark yellow with black spots.
3. Frons dark black.
4. Flagellar formula: L/W; ½ = 10/7.74; $^{2/2}$ = 7.74/7.74; $^{3/2}$ = 9.56/7.74; $^{4/2}$ = 37.5/7.74; $^{5/2}$ = 40/7.74; A = 2.70.
5. Anal appendages yellow with black tip.
6. Fore wing antenodal nervures 12 and postnodal nervures 9.
7. Hind wing antenodal nervures 9 and postnodal nervures 8.
8. Femora blackish with only four spines.
9. Tibia black with 9 spines.

Chapter 2

Biology of Dragonflies

Biology forms a basic information for the workers involved in biological control programmes for formulating mass rearing etc. (Sathe, 2004). Therefore, biology of a biocontrol agents has great importance.

In the life history of dragonflies there are three stages *i.e.* the egg, the larva and the adult. No pupal stage is present in dragonflies. But the change from larval to adult life is direct amphibiotic, that is, part of their life, the larval stage is passed in a watery environment and adults are terrestrial.

The Egg (Figure 50)

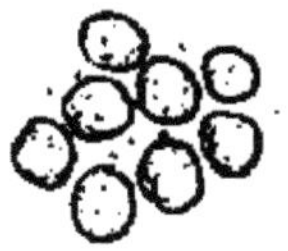

Figure 50: Life Cycle of Dragonfly: Eggs

The eggs are rounded or fusiform, and pale yellow in colour. In the zygoptera the eggs are deposited in the tissues of plants or in floating debris with the help of ovipositor. Generally they deposit on submerged or partially submerged objects, but several species oviposit in the tissues of plants, reeds or stems of plants, overhanging water, and at a height of several feet from the water's surface. In the Anisoptera the eggs are usually diposted straight into the water; a mass of eggs is exuded and stroked off by the insect rapidly skimming the water's surface, dipping its abdomen at intervals. Eggs are laid on reeds. However, some species oviposit in a similar manner to the Zygoptera, whilst some species deposit their eggs in the soil of gulleys. Later, they are washed down by a rains into water bodies. A third and more archaie, group of dragonflies deposit a mass of eggs on foliage overhanging the water, from whence the larvae descend down in water bodies as soon as they hatch out. Eggs hatch within few days to week.

The Larva (Figure 51)

The eggs hatch out as a tiny larvae enclosed in a thin membranous envelope which protect them until they find there watery environment, at least in the case of those which hatch out of water. This envelope is soon cast off, and the free-swimming larva or nymph makes its appearance. In different genera or species, but they all agree in possessing a highly specialized labium. This organ lies-flush beneath the head and thorax, and possesses, between the mentum and submentum, hinge at will by opening out. It is known as the mask and is employed in seizing its prey by means of the powerful hooks and jaws situated at its apex. The mask is variable in shape and importance in classification. In the Zygoptera the larvae are usually elongate, cylindrical, and possess two or three lamellar caudal gills. In some genera (of zygoptera only) they possess also pairs of so-called abdominal gills, which are, however, employed solely for the purpose of anchoring the surface of rocks or stones in swiftly flowing torrential streams. In general, the nymphs contain a pair of short antennae, three pairs of walking legs and developing wing pads (Figure 52) on the thorax as prominent appendages. Nymphal stage lasts for 3 months to 3 years.

Adults (Figure 52)

The adult insect shows a head, a prothorax, thorax and abdomen. The thorax carrying 3 pair of legs and 2 pairs of wings. The abdomen composed of ten segments, and carrying the genitalia of the male on the 2nd, 9th and 10th segments and appendages for seizing the female on the anal end of the 10th.

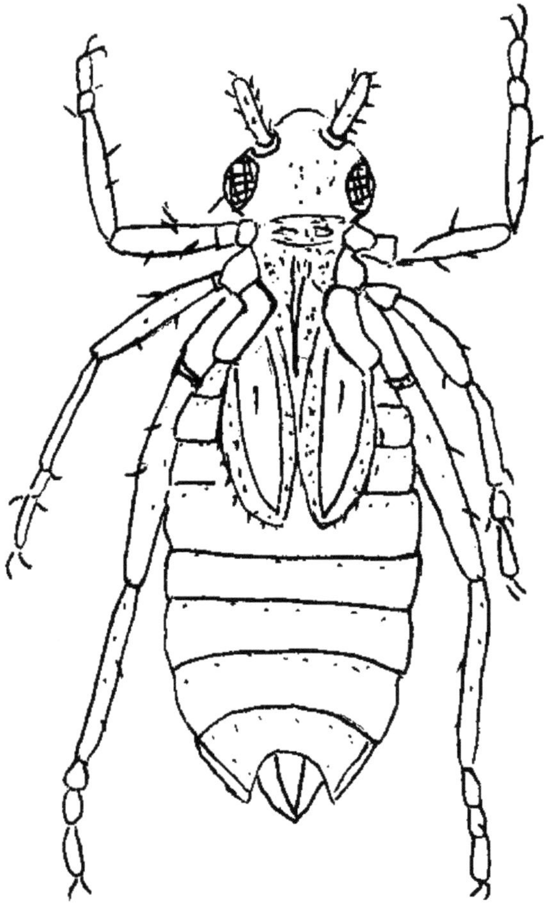

Figure 51: Life Cycle of Dragonfly: Nymph

The structure, function, biology, life history, taxonomy of these insects have been thoroughly worked out. The environmental bioassys evaluation, immunological, biochemical studies, behaviour, ecology, emergence, adaptation and their functional role in the environment, have also studied by some workers (Andrew and Tembhare, 1997; Andrew 2002; Andrew and Tembhare 1994; Andrew and Tembhare 1993; Andrew and Tembhare 1996; Atkin, 1980, Cannings *et al.*, 1991, Corbet, 1662, Corbet 1980, Corbet 1999;

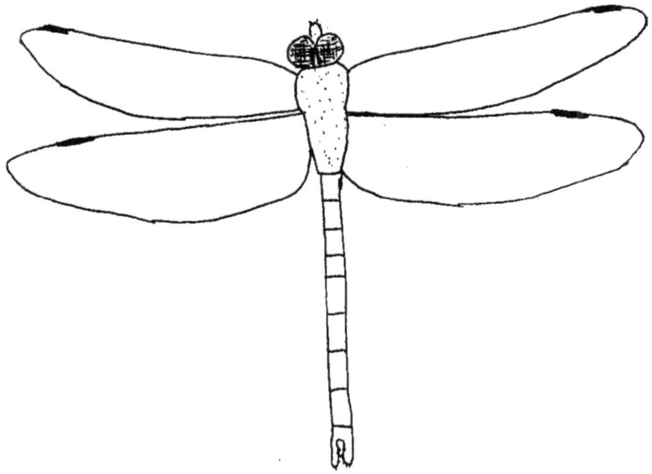

Figure 52: Life Cycle of Dragonfly: Adult

Dasgupta, 1957; Fraser, 1921c, Tembhare and Thakare 1977, Tembhare, 1979; Tembhare *et al.*, 1980; Tillyard, 1916, Wright, 1932; Kiauta, 1975 etc.).

Feeding and reproductive behaviour of Odonates are unique among animal taxa. Adult dragonflies prey upon small insects *viz.* mosquitoes, moths, jassids, midges, aphids etc. which are caught by anteriorly, directed prehensile forelegs. Larval feeding behaviour is very interesting. Larva remains motionless until a prey is detected by sight or touch. As soon as the prey comes near and within the range, the larva quickly extends its labial mask, grabs the prey and draws it back but slowly to the mandibles. The larvae feed on fish spawn, fish fry, fingerlings, mosquito larvae, mayfly nymphs, zooplankton tadpole etc.

As adult dragonflies prey upon adult mosquitoes, jassids, moths and allies and larval forms feed on mosquito larvae, they have been successfully employed in Biological control of mosquitoes in Myanmar (Burma) and paddy pests in Indonesia (Sathe, 2006). The larvae are voracious predators attacking only moving prey and have high preference for microcrustacea and other aquatic insects. Dragonfly nymphs consumed at least 30 per cent of their own body weight in a day.

Dragonflies are popularly supposed to sting, but in reality they are perfectly harmless insects, and the forceps which adorn the end of the abdomen are merely accessory sexual appendages; beyond their great powers of flight they have no defensive appliances. Thus, dragonflies do not bite or sting to man.

Economically dragonflies have great importance in destroying noxious pests like flies, mosquitoes and smaller moths. Some species which take to the wing only after dark or at dusk which live entirely on mosquitoes. A vast number of dragonflies are acting as scavengers of the atmosphere.

Dragonflies have but few enemies. They themselves, are the enemies since there is cannibalism in both in the larval and imaginal stages. Certain species, such as *Orthetrum sabina*, live almost exclusively upon their own kind, haunting the margins of tanks and lakes, where they make a rich living off the smaller fry. Birds, lizards, fishes, frogs and spiders are the potential enemies of dragonflies. Birds take a heavy toll of these insects during their emergence, when their weak flight makes them fall as easy prey to swallows, martins, minas and kingcrows. Lizards attack those species which are given to alighting on the ground. Fishes and frogs feed on odonates both during the larval and early imaginal stages. Tillyard mentions the finding of as many as thirty five undigested heads of the dragonflies in the stomach of a single trout.

Spiders and Mantids play but a small part in this respect, and it is extremely rare to find a dragonfly caught up in a spiders web. Tillyard mentions that large numbers of the smaller species are caught by the Giant Sundew of Australia (*Drosera binata*), also it has been noted the case of *Ishnura delicata* and the common Indian sundew, *Drosera pellata*.

Dragonflies are attacked by few parasites either as larvae or as the imago. Several species of small Hymenoptera (Trichogrammidae and Myrmaridae) deposit their eggs in those of dragonflies. A small nematode is found in the gut of the imago. Gregarines occupy the same situation in the larvae of dragonflies.

The symbiosis are known with dragonflies. A small red mite (a Hydrachnid) is commonly found clinging to the wings, legs and thorax of certain species, specially of *Ceriagrion coromandelianum* and species of *Sympetrum* of temperate climates; these attach themselves to the insects at the time of emergence as a means of dispersal to other localities. It is unknown why certain species only are thus employed as living aeroplanes, but the fact remains. Another form of symbiosis is met with in certain larvae which become coated with dense masses of algae, which protect them effectually from their enemies and prey alike.

Migration is also characteristic of dragonflies. Migratory flight is usually in a direction from east to west, but during October and November vast number of the smaller species may be seen flying northwards up the West coast, their emergence appearing to coincide with the draining of paddy lands prior to the harvest. This behaviour is managed in pest control strategies.

Dragonflies cling with remarkable tenacity to their watery birth places and although on emergence they wander a far, they return to their former homes for purposes of breeding; males indeed rarely depart from such places, but await the return of the females over ponds and streams. The number of males are vastly exceeds the number of females. *Anaciaceschna martini* mating takes place in the forest or away from water. This order of preponderance is reversed.

Since dragonflies breed in water, it happens that the number of species found bears a direct ratio to the rainfall or water supplies of any particular district. So far as India concerned the Western Ghats, the southern slopes of the Himalayas, and the wet tracts of Myanmar and ShriLanka are richest in species. The drier zones are not without dragonflies but, have their own distinctive fauna.

Some dragonfly species found confined to a very short stretch of river or a small patch of marshy lands in the forest. *Chloroneura apicalis* has been found only on a short stretch of the Cauvery River of Fraserpet.

Dragonflies are very seasonal. In India the best months for collecting dragonflies are May and June and September to the first half of November, that is, during the months which precede and follow the South-west monsoon. Common species are not only widely distributed but occur nearly the whole year round. Quite a number of species are strictly confined to certain attitudes, a zone lying between 2,000 and 3,500 feet yielding the richest fauna. The hot plains appear to be inimical to these and to act as a barrier to their spread; this isolated mountain groups have developed a peculiar fauna of their own resembling islands in this respect.

The Indian odonate fauna has borrowed largely from Malaysia and to a less extent, from the Palearctic, but it is rich in entogenic groups, the origin of some of which is decidedly obscure. The chain of the Western Ghats has a rich fauna, many forms which are entirely restricted to it. A few Ethiopian and Australian forms have made their way to India; examples of such are *Zygonyx torrida isis* from the former and *Hemicordulia asiatica* from the latter.

A dragonfly after emergence takes several days to develop its fall colours and become fully chitinized, that is, hardened. Thus a newly fledged insect will not only be poor in colouring, but will also shrivel up after death and make an unsightly specimen. The larvae of many species are frequently dredged up, the imagines of which have never been seen in that particular neighbourhood. Other species depart into the heart of the jungle directly after emergence, and are never seen from that time onwards. This particularly related to the females and to the Gomphinae.

The aquatic life of larvae varies greatly in length, that of the genus *Lestes* being probably the shortest about three months in all. The larger species take from one to 3 years to reach maturity. Riverine larvae are the most difficult to rear, as they need running water in which to develop. Odonates are cannibalistic forms. Therefore, it is very necessary to keep them apart or the numbers will be found to diminish with alarming rapidity. For the most part, they feed on their own kind, but tadpoles, small fishes and the larvae of many flies or caddisflies forms a suitable diet.

The adults must be netted in the same way as butterflies and no special modification need be made on this method. The eyesight of a dragonfly is remarkable acute. It is best to strike from below, as their sight is less acute from that angle.

Some species found resting on rocks in mid-stream, or perched on herbage protostictas and platystictas rests on weedy banks of tanks, ponds or lakes, or in the shallows of drying streams. The smaller species are found and on account of their minute size and slow movements they must be sought for carefully. Many species may be taken by sweeping the net amongst rank herbage.

In the dark undergrowth of jungles many of the smaller genera, such as *Copera, Platycnemis* and *Mortonagrion,* are only found in such habitats. Many species prefer open country and will be found resting on bare patches of ground.

The IUCN/SCC Odonata specialist group (Moore, 1977) has prepared a Dragonfly Action Plan to address the problems, which threaten dragonflies and make recommendations to conserve them. The plan focuses on the importance of creating protected areas such as nature reserves and conserving important habitats. The Action Plan also contained lists of dragonflies considered to be priority species for further study and conservation action. The priority species from the oriental region are listed below:

Priority Species (based on recommendations of the IUCN/SCC, Odonata Specialists Group, Moore, 1997).

Suborder	*Family*	*Species*	*Distribution*
Anisozygoptera	Epiophlebiidae		
		Epiophlebia superstes (Selys, 1889)	Japan
		Epiophlebia laidlawi Tillyard, 1921	India, Nepal
Zygoptera	Calopterggidae		
		Noguchiphaea yoshikoae Asahina, 1976	Thailand
		Caliphaca confusa Hagen in Selys, 1859	Bhutan, China, India Laos, Myanmar, Nepal
		Caliphaca consimilis McLachlan, 1894	China, (Guangxi, Sichuan, Yunnan and Zhejiana)
		Caliphaca thailandica Asahina 1976	Thailand
		Diphlebiidae philoganga loringae Fraser, 1927	Myanmar, Thailand
		Philoganga montana (Hagen in Selys, 1859)	Bangladesh, India, Malaysia, Nepal
		Philogana robusta Navas, 1936	China
		Philoganga vetusta Ris, 1912.	China, Hongkong

Contd...

Contd...

Suborder	Family	Species	Distribution
Megapodagrionidae			
		Lestomima flavastigma May, 1933	China
		Rhipidolestes aculeatus Ris, 1912	China
		Rhipidolestes alleni Wilson, 2000.	(Taiwan) Japan
		Rhipidolestes apicatus Navas 1934	China (Guangxi) China (Zhejiang)
		Rhipidolestes asatoi Asahima, 1994	Japan (Kyushu)
		Rhipidolestes bastiaani Zhu and Yang, 1998	China (Shaanxi)
		Rhipidolestes cyanoflavus Wilson, 2000	China (Guangdong)
		Rhipidolestes hiraoi Yamamoto, 1955	Japan (Shikoku)
		Rhipidolestes janetae Wilson, 1997	China (Hongkong)
		Rhipidolestes jucundus Lieftinck, 1948	China (Fujian)
		Rhipidolestes malaisei Lieftinck, 1948	Myanmar
		Rhipidolestes rectans (Needham, 1929)	China (Zhejiang)
		Rhipidolestes okinawanus Asahina, 1951	Japan (Okinawa)
		Rhipidolestes owadai Asahima, 1997	Vietnam
		Rhipidolestes rubripes (Navas, 1936)	China (Jiangxi)
		Rhipidolestes truncatidens Schmidt, 1931	China (Fujian, Guangdong)
		Rhipidolestes yangbingi Davies, 1998	China (Sichuan)
		Devadatta argyoides (Selys, 1959)	Indonesia, Myanmar, Singapore, Thialand

Contd...

Contd...

Suborder	*Family*	*Species*	*Distribution*
		Devadatta ducatrix Lieftinck, 1969	China (Guangxi) Vietnam
		Devadatta multinervosa Fraser, 1933	Laos
		Devadatta podolestoides Laidlaw, 1934	Indonesia and Malaysia (Borneo)
		Philosina buchi Ris 1917	China (Fujian, Guanglong, Guangxi)
		Philosina alba Wilson 1999	China (Guanglong, Hainan)
	Pseudolestidae		
		Pseudolestes mirabilis Kirby, 1900	China (Hainan)
Anisoptera	Onychothemistinae		
		Onychothemis abnormis Brauer, 1968	Indonesia, Philippines
		Onychothemis celebensis Ris 1912	Indonesia, (Celebes)
		Onychothemis coccinea Lieftinck 1953	Indonesia, Malaysia
		Onychothemis culminicola Forster, 1904	Indonesia, Malaysia, Manmar, Thailand
		Onychothemis testaceab Laidlaw, 1902	China (Guangdong, Guangxi, Hainan, Hong kong, Taiwan) Indonesia, Malaysia, Myanmar, Srilanka, Thailand, Vietnam

Contd...

Contd...

Suborder	*Family*	*Species*	*Distribution*
2. Monotypic Genera from the Oriental Region (Genera containing only one species)			
Zygoptera	Megapodagrionidae		
		Agriomorpha fusca May, 1933	China (Guangdong, Guangxi, Hainan, Hong Kong)
	Synlestidae		
		Sinolestes editus Needham, 1930	China (Fujian, Guangdong, Guangxi and Zhejiang)
Anisoptera	Gomphidae		
		Gastrogomphus abdominalis (McLachlan, 1884)	China
		Labrogomphus torvus Needham, 1931	China (Guangdong, Guangxi, Hainan, Hong Kong)
3. Dragonflies with unusual biology from the Oriental Region			
Zygoptera	Coeagrionidae		
		Mortonagrion hiroselb Asahima, 1971	China (Hong kong) Japan (Salt tolerant species found to associate with *Phragmites* sp. reed).

Chapter 3

Utilization in Biological Pest Control Programme

Introduction

Dragonflies are ideal predators of many insect pests and have an important role in biological pest control in various agroecosystems and forest ecosystems. About 6500 species of dragonflies are known from all over the world (Kakkassery, 2003). From India about 600 species have been reported (Sathe and Shinde, 2006a).

Dragonflies and damselflies have proved to be the potential biocontrol agents of mosquitoes and rice pests all around the world. However, from India, very little attention is paid on this important group of insects with respect to its utility in biological control of insect pests (Sathe, 2005). In past, van vredon and Ahmadsabidi (1986), Thomas *et al.* (1988), Kakkassery (2004), Sathe (2005), Sathe *et al.* (2006), etc. attempted studies related to biological pest control using dragonflies.

Materials and Methods

For rearing of dragonflies following materials are adopted.

Materials

Glass Cages (Figure 53 and 54)

Two types of glass cages (Figures 53 and 54) are used for handling dragonflies. Both cages are quadrangular in shape with size 25 x 25 x 30 cm. Each cage consists wooden case and glass walls on all sides. In first type (Figure 53) door side is closed by muslin cloth with a sleeve for handling the insects. The door is prepared with glass in the second type (Figure 54).

Glass Troughs (Figure 55)

The glass troughs (size 9 x 20, 12 x 25 cm) are to be used for rearing of nymphs of dragonflies collected from different natural habitat. The glass troughs are covered with muslin cloth for protection and prevention of escape of adult dragonflies.

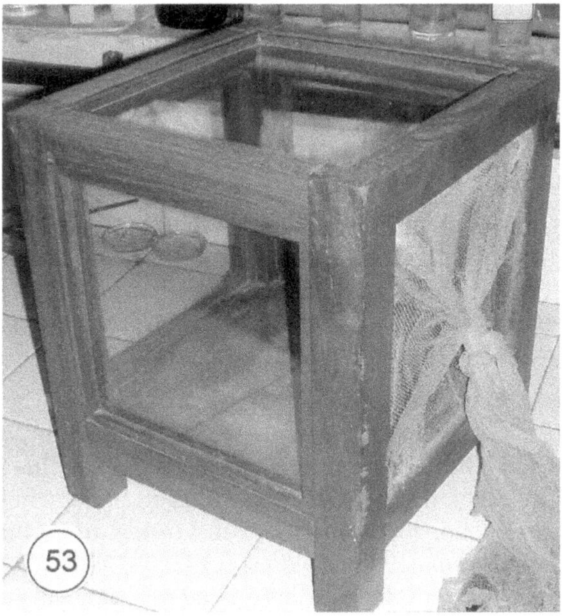

Figure 53

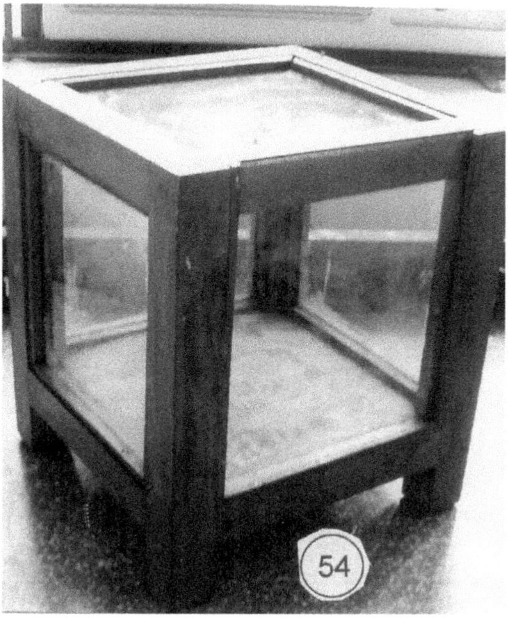

Figure 54

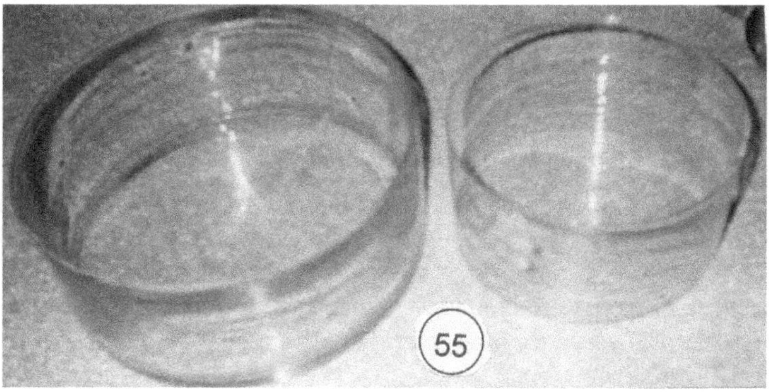

Figure 55

Plastic Containers

Plastic containers of size 18 x 6 cm, 13 x 5 cm, 12.5 x 4.5 cm and 4 x 4 cm in diameter and height respectively are to be used for rearing the nymphs (naids) and handling the insects.

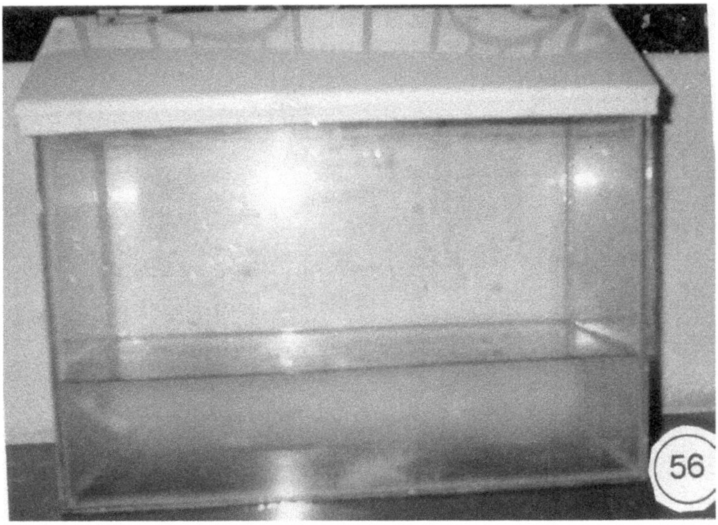

Figure 56

Aquarium (Figure 56)

Glass aquarium of size 46 cm x 20.5 cm x 30 cm in length width and height respectively with a iron slanting door is to be used for rearing the nymphs of dragonflies.

Methods

Collection of Nymphs and Dragonflies

Nymphs of dragonflies are collected from various aquatic habitats and / or from Koyna Dam and around area of Western Ghats of Satara district and reared in aquarium (Figure 56) in the laboratory on natural food material for adult emergence. The adults, thus formed are to be considered for mass rearing of the species and taxonomical description

Collection of Larvae/Nymphs (Naids) in Biodiversity Studies

The nymphs are collected by sweeping aquatic habitats with the help of dip net. Anisoptera larvae are to be kept in containers with a bit of wet moss or other vegetation to keep the humidity high and to develop them in the media.

Exuviae (cast larval skins) are also collected from aquatic plants, rocks, logs and other supports. The exuviae are dried and pinned through the base of the wing cases and placed a small drop of white glue at the point where the pin exited the base of thorax ventrally. Some times the exuvae are also preserved in 70 per cent alcohol.

Adults

A long handled aerial net is used for collecting adult dragonflies. A net opening of atleast 18" is taken. The nets are of three kinds *i.e.* black net, white net and green net based on colour of mesh. However, white nets are used for collection of dragonfly adults. They are easier to find the specimen in the net. A wide wesh (but small enough to hold the smallest specimens) is preferred because this reduces air resistance and allow a faster swing. Swing at fast-flying agile species from behind as they fly by many will be easy to catch by this insect net.

After capturing the adult specimen, they are placed in a glassine envelope (available in several sizes- the most versatile is 3.5"x2.25"– at stamp collector stores). The wings should be together above the back. In general, only one specimen is kept in each envelope.

Dragonflies damage each other hence, they are placed for some time in pairs caught in tandem or in copula in the same envelope. The large sized specimen are placed single in the single envelope, keeping away from each. The collection number (cross-referenced to field notes) or full collection data is written on the envelope by soft pencil, India ink or other ink which is in soluble in acetone.

Teneral (recently emerged) adults are fragile and preserved poorly. They are placed in paper bags for a day or two for handing of cuticle and for colour development of patterns. The emerging adults are placed in a bag and the associated exuviate are kept and cross-referenced for adult specimen.

Preparation of Adults

The envelopes containing line dragonflies are kept cool as possible in field collection and transfer. They are stored in a non-crushable box. This allowed the specimens to empty their digestive tracts. Colour is usually preserved better in a specimen with an empty gut. The colour pattern of some species, especially some blue ones (*e.g. Aeshna* spp.) are faded soon after capture. This fading can often be reversed by exposing the specimen to sunlight. However, such species are treated in acetone immediately.

Methods of Biocontrol of Pests

There are four methods of biological control of insects pests.

1. Collection and destruction of pests by keeping labour (control by man as biocontrol agent).
2. Collection of dragonflies and damselflies from natural habitat and releasing them in a target area with appropriate density.
3. Mass rearing of dragonflies and releasing them in target area for pest suppression.
4. Importation of dragonfly species, their mass rearing and field release for suppression of pests.

Mostly second and third methods are used in biological pest control since they are viable and easy to do. In second method habitat identification of dragonflies has tremendous importance since one can easily collect the dragonflies for sending them to other target areas for pest control. This is easy method and required no laboratory work and technical man power.

Third method need technical skill and knowledge of rearing of pests and dragonfly species and need good laboratories for rearing. In fact, mass rearing is soul of biocontrol programme. Thus, rearing counts the success of the control programme.

Mass Rearing of Dragonflies

Mass rearing techniques for dragonflies have been developed previously by Mac Neil (1952), Fonseka (2000) and Silsby (2001). The latest trends of rearing of dragonflies given by Fonseka (2000) and Silsby (2001) are quite familiar to workers in biological pest control. However, the present methodology is modification of existing one and standardized for rearing dragonfly species. The rearing of dragonflies is divided into some special steps which are given below.

During the first step of rearing, eggs of the females are to be collected from natural environment (habitat). Dragonfly females lay their eggs into water. Neting the females is best way of collecting eggs. Tip of the abdomen of collected female is to be dipped in the water in small petridish. The female will start egg laying in the water. However, the eggs of females can also be collected by watching females in the field when they lay eggs on plants in case of damselflies.

Food for Nymphs

The best food for the young ones of dragonflies is paramoecium which can be easily cultured and prepared by putting some hay in the water for 3-5 days. Newly hatched nymphs should be immediately transferred by pipette into small jars which contain a little duck weed, *Lemna* for aeration, and provided with paramoecium as food for first instars. However, chief losses occur at 3rd and 4th instars. The nymphs grow fairly faster and 4th and 5th instars should be transferred to large jars or small aquariums. In addition to duckweed a little *Vallisneria* should be introduced into aquarium for aeration. 5th instars are given *Daphnia* and *Cyclops* in sufficient quantity for feeding. Later, some nymphs are separated and kept in larger aquarium for avoiding cannibalism amongst the dragonfly nymphs and for avoiding crowding. Approaching maturity, the nymphs are fed with mosquito larvae or red worms. While, the 7th and onward nymphs are provided with mudworms, tubifers, etc. However, maturing nymphs are separated into large aquarium. In this stage, the aquarium must have reeds for climbing the nymphs upon them and thus, facilitating nymphs to attach their exuvie for becoming adults. For preventing excape (flight) of the newly emerged adults, a musclin-cloth cover should be used to aquarium. Thus, after getting sufficient number of adults (mass reared), they are released into the target area with appropriate density and at appropriate time against target pest species. Mass reared dragonflies are to be released in the field by two ways.

Inoculative Release

This refers to small scale release (10, 20, 50, 100, 200).

Inductive Release

This refers to large scale release (with large number) (500, 750, 1000, 5000).

Trials in Kolhapur Region

Release of Dragonflies in Mulberry Ecosystem

A mulberry plot of one acre is to be selected. The plot is kept control (no pesticides is treated and weekly observations are made on the availability of dragonflies, damselflies and their predatory feeding behaviour with respect to mulberry pests, specially, syntomids, cutworms, defoliators, jassids, leaf roller and stem borers at morning hours 8.30 a.m. to 9.30 a.m. Later, the dragonflies and damselflies feeding on the above pests have been collected with the help of insect net and identified by consulting literature (Fraser 1933, 1934, 1936, 1957; Kulkarni and Prasad, 2002; Lahiri, 1987; Prasad, 1995, 1996, 1999; Prasad and Varshney, 1995; Prasad and Kulkarni, 2002; Silsby 2001 etc.).

20 individuals of dragonflies are introduced in one acre mulberry field of Kolhapur and observations are made on population of mulberry jassids on sticky papers (size A-4). Five such papers are to be installed in plot. One at centre and other four at four corners at height of 3½ feet and number of jassids sticked to the paper surface are to be counted at one week interval.

During the survey studies following dragonflies/damselflies were found feeding on various mulberry pests. Their abundance and prey are mentioned in Table 2.

Table 2: Dragonflies/Damselflies Feeding on Mulberry Pests and their Abundance

Sl.No.	*Dragonfly/Damselfly*	*Rice Pests*	*Abundance*
1.	*Diplacodes trivialis* (Rambur)	Sylepta, Moths	Common
2.	*Neurothermis tullia tullia* (Drury)	Jassids, moths	Dominant
3.	*Crocothemis servilia* (Drury)	Moths, Jassids	Dominant
4.	*Brachythemis contaminate* (Fabr.)	Moths	Dominant
5.	*Orthetrum sabina sabina* (Drury)	Jassids, leaf roller	Dominant
6.	*Trithemis aurora* (Burmeister)	Jassids, moths	Common
7.	*Pantala flaviscens* (Fabricius)	Jassids, leaf eaters, thrips	Dominant
8.	*Rhyothemis v. variegata* (Linnaeus)	Moths, Jassids, Thrips, aphids	Common
9.	*Ishnura delicata*	Jassids	Common
10.	*I. senegalensis*	Moths, jassids, spiders	Common
11.	*Bradinopyga germinata*	Jassids, midge, mosquitoes	Common
12.	*Pontamarcha conger*	Jassids, moths	Common

Out of 27 species of Odonates *C. servilia* and *C. flaviscens* were most dominant in the mulberry agroecosystem of Kolhapur district, India. The above two species, significantly reduced the population of jassids. Several species of Odonates (Table 1) found feeding on jassids and lepidopteran pests in the field of mulberry in Kolhapur.

During years 2005-06 jassid catches on sticky papers after introduction of 20 dragonflies (10 c.s. and 10 c.f.) per week showed significant reduction in jassid population in Kolhapur region.

Mass rearing and release of predators proved worthy in pest management in mulberry agro-ecosystem (Sathe and Mulla, 1999). Sometimes cannibalism among the members of the same predatory species possess a problem. Therefore, conservation of natural enemies in situ is a feasible option. Dragonflies and damselflies are amongst the most conspicuous predators of insect pests with irrigated fields. Hence, they should be utilized in mulberry pest control.

Nymphs of dragonflies and damselflies feed on larvae of mosquitoes and midges in aquatic habitat and adults consume moths of *Spodoptera litura, Sylepta derogata, Spilosoma obliqua* and leafhoopers (Jassids). From Orissa and Assam (India) Krishnaswamy *et al.* (1984) recorded *Ceriagrion coromandelianum* (Fabr.) feeding on yellow stem borer *Scirpophaga incertulus* (Wlk.) and leaf folder *Cnaphalocrocis medinalis* (Linn.). It also feed on nymphs and adults of white backed plant hopper *Sogatella furcifera* (Horvath) while, *C. pygmaea* (Ramb.) suppressed the population of yellow stem borer and leaf folder moths in addition to the nymphs and adults of green leaf hoppers in rice fields of Orissa.

Israel and Padmanabhan (1976) demonstrated the role of *Ictinogomphus rapax* (Ramb.) in controlling adults of yellow stem borer and leaf folders in rice field of Orissa. They also assessed potential of *Urothemis signata* (Ramb.) and *Orthetrum sabina* (Drury) against adults of yellow stem borer and leaf folders on rice crop in Orissa. Further, they reported suppression of population of caseworm of rice due to the introduction of *Diaplacodes nebulosa* (Fbr.) and *Pantala flaviscens* (Fbr.). The above Odonates have been utilized by Krishnaswamy *et al* (1984).

Bharadwaj and Pawar (1987) reported *Ischnura* feeding on rice pests from Chattisgarh region of India in 1987. Israel and Padmanabhan recorded 14 species of Odonates suppressing the rice pest populations in rice agroecosystems of Assam, Orissa and Madhya Pradesh. The pest predatory Odonates refers to *C. coromandelianum, A. pygmaea, I. delicata, I. rofostigma, Ictinogomphus rapax, U. signata, O. sabina, Pontamarcha abscura, Brachythemis contaminata, A. panorpoides, D. trivialis, D. nebulosa, T. pallidinervis, R. variegata* and *P. flaviscens*. Inspite of much more biodiversity of dragonflies in Western Maharashtra no attention was paid on the utility of dragonflies in biological pest control of mulberry pests. Secondly, there is no any account of predatory dose for controlling pests in the Indian fields.

Decrease in the population of lepidopterous pests on mulberry crop was noted by spot observations and collection of moths within one hour by 1 man search. Although it is necessary to adopt effective sampling method for mulberry pests and biological control of mulberry pests.

Dragonflies and damselflies are potential biocontrol agents of several mulberry pests and need their mass production and their utilization in biological control of mulberry pests.

Release of Dragonflies in Paddy Fields of Kolhapur

A paddy plot of 1 acre was selected in the field of Kolhapur. The plot was kept control (no pesticides were treated) and weekly observations were made on the availability of dragonflies, damselflies, and their predatory feeding behaviours with respect to rice pests specially, stem borers, leaf rollers and plant hoppers at morning hours 8.30 am to 9.30 am. Later, the dragonflies and damselflies feeding on the above pests have been collected with the help of insect net and identified by consulting literature.

20 individuals of dragonflies 10 *C. servilia* and 10 *P. flaviscens* have been introduced in one acre paddy field of Kolhapur (Panchgaon) and observations were made on population of brown plant hopper *Nilaparvata lugens* (Stal.) on sticky papers (size 27 cm x 38 cm). Five such papers have been installed in one acre plot, one at centre and other four corners at the height of 3½ ft and number of brown plant hoppers sticked to paper surface have been counted at one week interval.

During the survey studies, following dragonflies/damselflies were found feeding on various rice pests. Their abundance and preys are mentioned in Table 3.

Table 3: Dragonflies/Damselflies Feeding on Rice Pests and their Abundance

Sl.No.	*Dragonfly/Damselfly*	*Rice Pests*	*Abundance*
1.	*Diplacodes trivialis* (Rambur)	Moths	Common
2.	*D. nebulosa* (Fabricius)	Borers (Moths)	Common
3.	*Neurothermis tullia tullia* Drury	Jassids, moths	Dominant
4.	*Crocothemis servilia* Drury	Borers	Dominant
5.	*Brachythemis contaminata* (Fabr.)	Moths	Common
6.	*Orthetrum sabina sabina* (Drury)	Borers, leaf roller	Dominant
7.	*O. chrysis* Selys	Pyralids	Dominant
8.	*Acisoma P. panurpoides* Rambur	Moths	Rare
9.	*Trithemis aurora* (Burmeister)	Jassids	Common
10.	*Pantala flaviscens* (Fabricius)	Borers, jassids leaf eaters	Dominant
11.	*Rhyothemis v. variegata* (Linnaeus)	Moths	Common
12.	*Ceriagrion coromandelianum*	Jassids	Rare
13.	*Agriocnemis* sp.	Jassids	Dominant
14.	*Lestes elata*	Moths, leaf hoppers	Dominant
15.	*Ishnura delicata*	Jassids	Dominant
16.	*I. senegalensis*	Jassids, spider	Dominant

Out of 16 species of Odonates *C. servilia* and *C. flaviscens* were most dominant in the rice agroecosystem of Kolhapur district, India. The above two species significantly reduced the population of BPH (Brown plant hopper), *Nilaparvata lugens* (Stal.). Several species of Odonates (Table 3) found feeding on WBPH, Green leaf hoppers and lepidopteran pests in the field of paddy in Kolhapur. The performance of *C. servilia* and *P. flaviscens* for suppression of BPH is shown in Table 4.

Mass rearing and release of above two predators proved worthy in pest management in rice agro-ecosystem (Van Vredan and Ahmadazabidi, 1986, Sathe 2005). They also feed on nymphs and adults of white backed plant hopper *Sogatella furcifera* (Horvath). While, *C. pygmaea* (Ramb.) suppressed the population of yellow stem borer and leaf folder moths in addition to the nymphs and adults of green leaf hoppers in rice fields in Orissa.

Table 4: Average (Year 2003-05) Brown Plant Hopper (BPH) Catches on Sticky Papers After Introduction of 20 Dragonflies (10 C.S. and 10 C.F.) per Week

Weeks	*Sticky Paper-I*	*Sticky Paper-II*	*Sticky Paper-III*	*Sticky Paper-IV*	*Sticky Paper-V*	*Average*
July 1st	1112	1132	1044	1119	1122	1105.80
IInd	1023	982	992	1003	1007	1001.40
IIIrd	810	840	795	888	901	846.80
IVth	620	607	590	578	720	623.00
Aug. 1st	611	549	504	449	423	507.00
IInd	492	412	419	392	314	405.80
IIIrd	369	362	355	340	302	345.60
IVth	159	132	148	102	215	151.20
July Control Average	1320	1242	1248	1347	1369	1305.20
August Control Average	1207	1222	1201	1321	1105	1213.20

In paddy field a constant number, 20 species of dragonflies (1:1, Cs: Pf) have been released per week and BPH (plant hopper) have been accounted on sticky (greasy) papers. The number of plant hoppers was decreased from 1305.20 to 151.20 individuals on each sticky paper within two moths (July–Aug.) showing the significant role of dragonflies, *C. servilia* and *C. flaviscens* in suppression of jassid populations on rice crop.

Decrease in the population of lepidopterous pests in rice crop was noted by spot observations and collection of moths within one hour by 1 man search.

Conclusion

1. Dragonflies and Damselflies are potential biocontrol agents of several pests of paddy and mulberry and need their mass production and utilization in biological control programmes of pests in India.
2. Odonata biocontrol agents help in reducing the load of pesticides on mulberry and rice agroecosystems and high risk of pesticides to humans.

3. Biological pest control programmes should be encouraged in paddy and mulberry ecosystems in India.

Dragonflies for Controlling Mosquitoes

Mosquitoes are responsible for causing fetal diseases such as Malaria, Filariasis, Dengue, Japanese encepalitis, Chikungunia etc. to human being. Their control with pesticides is difficult due to resistance against pesticides. Therefore, controlling mosquitoes by biological means is ecofriendly and permanent method of pest control. Mosquitoes have been controlled by using dragonflies in several countries of the world.

According to Corbet (1999), there are two approaches to the biological control of mosquitoes namely inoculation and augmentative release (AR). Both approaches are useful for mosquito control. Under inoculative release natural enemies of pests are introduced into an environment where they are not already present, during which enemies multiply naturally until they reach a level such that they either eliminate the pest or keep the pest population down to a level of deemed acceptable to humans. However, this method has limited success. Augmentative release can be highly successful since this method entails prior estimation of the number of natural enemies needed to active suppression to required level and then realizing sufficient number into a closed system. Augmentative release is practiced routinely in several countries for suppression of pests in green house, close environment from which either biocontrol agent nor pest can disperse. Odonata in general are predators of several insects. Amongst their preys, houseflies and mosquitoes are prominently predated (Metcalf and Flint, 1979). Thomas *et al* (1988) studied predatory efficiency of nymphs of *Bradinophyga jaminata* and *Brachythemis contaminata* on mosquito larvae. They found that these Odonates were good predators of mosquito larvae.

In Cuba, Santhamarina and Mijares (1986) made field and laboratory observations to study the efficacy of nymphs of anisopterans such as *Pantala flavescens, Tramea abdominalis* and proved them good predators of *Culex quinquefaciatus.*

A sizable work has been made from Japan in connection with the control of various types of mosquito larvae. Urabe *et al.* (1986) studied and evaluated the predatory capacity and efficiency of

Table 5: Dragonfly Pest Predator Index

Sl.No.	Dragonfly Species	Prey		Occurrence
		Common Name	Scientific Name	
	ZYGOPTERA (DAMSELFLIES)			
	FAMILY (OENAGRIDAE)			
1.	*Lestes viridulus* (Rambur)	Moth	*Chilo suppressalis* (Walk)	Common
2.	*Lestes praemorsa* Selys	Moth	*C. suppressalis* (Walk)	Rare
3.	*Lestes elata* Hagen	Leaf hopper	*Nephotettix virescens* (Distant)	Common
4.	*Lestes malabarica* Fraser	Leaf hopper	*N. virescens*	Rare
5.	*Lestes nodalis* Selys	Leaf hopper	*N. virescens*	Rare
6.	*Lestis umbrinus* Selys	Moth	*Scirpophaga incertulus* (Walk)	Common
7.	*Ceylonolestes pulcherrima* (Fraser)	Moth	Unknown pyralid	Rare
8.	*Copera marginipes* (Rambur)	Rice moth	*Proceras indicus* Kapur	Rare
9.	*Copera vittata* (Selys)	Rice moth	*P. indicus*	Common
10.	*Caconeura verticalls verticalls* Selys	Rice jassid	*N. virescens*	Rare
11.	*Caconeura ramburi* (Fraser)	Rice jassid	*N. virescens*	Common
12.	*Caconeura risi* (Fraser)	Rice moth	*C. suppressalis*	Common
13.	*Caconeura sita* Kirby	Rice moth	*C. suppressalis*	Rare
14.	*Disparoneura quadrimaculata* Rambur	Diamond back moth	*Plutella xylostella* (Lin.)	Common

Contd...

Table 5–Contd...

Sl.No.	*Dragonfly Species*	*Prey*		*Occurrence*
		Common Name	*Scientific Name*	
15.	*Disparoneura souteri* Fraser	Diamond back moth	*P. xylostella*	Common
16.	*Disparoneura nigerrima* Laidlaw	Cotton jassid	*Empoasca devastans* Distant	Rare
17.	*Chloroneura quadrimaculata*	Paddy hopper	*Sogatella furcifera* (Hrvath)	Common
18.	*Indoneura ramburi* Fraser	Caster capsule-borer	*Dichocrocis punctiferalis* Guenee	Common
19.	*Indoneura risi* Fraser	Caster jassid	*Empoasca binota* Pruthi	Common
20.	*Melanoneura bilineata* Fraser	Moth	Unknown pyralid moth	Rare
21.	*Esme cyaneovittata* Fraser	Midgefly	*Contarinia* sp.	Common
22.	*Esme mudiensis* Fraser	Jassid	*E. devastans*	Common
23.	*Phylloneura westermanni* (Selys)	Mosquito	*Culex* sp.	Common
24.	*Elattoneura tetrica* Laidlaw	Jassid	*S. furcifera*	Common
25.	*Pseudagrion microcephalum* (Ramb.)	Paddy moth	*Chilo infuscatellus* (Snell.)	Rare
26.	*Pseudagrion malabaricum* Fraser	Paddy moth	*C. infuscatellus*	Common
27.	*Pseudagrion decorum* (Rambur)	Rice moth	*S. incertulus*	Rare
28.	*Pseudagrion hypermelas* Selys	Rice moth	*S. incertulus*	Rare
29.	*Pseudagrion indicum* Fraser	Rice moth	*S. incertulus*	Rare

Contd...

Table 5–Contd...

Sl.No.	*Dragonfly Species*	*Prey*		*Occurrence*
		Common Name	*Scientific Name*	
30.	*Archibasis mimetes praeclara* Fraser	Mosquito	*Culex* sp.	Common
31.	*Archibasis oscillanus* (Selys)	Mosquito	*Anopheles, Culex*	Rare
32.	*Ceriagrion rubiae* Laidlaw	Mosquito	*Culex* sp.	Rare
33.	*Ceriagrion coromandelianum* (Fabr.)	Paddy jassid	*S. furcifera*	Common
34.	*Ceriagrion cerinorubellum* (Brauer)	Paddy jassid	*S. furcifera*	Common
35.	*Ceriagrion aurantiacum* (Laidlaw)	Paddy jassid	*S. furcifera*	Rare
36.	*Ceriagrion olivaceum* (Laidlaw)	Mango jassid	*Indioscopus* sp.	Rare
37.	*Aciagrion accidentale* (Laidlaw)	Moth	Pyralid moth	Common
38.	*Aciagrion hisopa* (Selys)	Moth	Unknown pyralid	Common
39.	*Aciagrion pallidum* (Selys)	Jassid	*Empoasca* sp.	Rare
40.	*Ichneura senegalensis* (Rambur)	Paddy jassid	*N. virescens*	Common
49.	*Enallagma parvum*	Mosquito	*Culex* sp.	Common
50.	*Cercion calamorum* (Ris)	Mosquito	*Culex* sp.	Rare
51.	*Mortonagrion varralli* Fraser	Midgefly	*Contarinia* sp.	Rare
52.	*Coenagrion dyeri* Fraser	Mosquito	*Culex* sp.	Common

Contd...

Table 5–Contd...

Sl.No.	*Dragonfly Species*	*Prey*		*Occurrence*
		Common Name	*Scientific Name*	
53.	*Onychargia* sp.	Moth	Pyraustid moth	Common
54.	*Prodasineura verticalis annandalei* Fraser	Mosquito	*Culex* sp.	Common
55.	*Esme cyaneovittata* Fraser	Paddy jassid	*N. virescens*	Not common
		FAMILY–AGRIDAE		
56.	*Colocypha laidlawi* (Fraser)	Mango jassid	*Indioscopus* sp.	Rare
57.	*Labellago lineata indica* (Fraser)	Moth	Pyraustid moth	Common
58.	*Indophaea dispar* (Rambur)	Mango jassid	*Indioscopus* sp.	Common
59.	*Indophaea cardinalis* (Fraser)	Psyllid	*Diphorina citri* K.	Common
60.	*Neurobasis chinensis chinensis*	White fly	*Dialeurodes* sp.	Rare
61.	*Vestalis gracillis gracillis* (Rambur)	Mango jassid	*Amritodus atkinsoni* Let.	Common
62.	*Vestalis apicalis apicalis* Selys	Jassid	*A. atkinsoni*	Rare
63.	*Onychargia atrocyana*	Mosquito	*Anopheles* sp.	Common
64.	*Protostica anelopoides* Fraser	Moth	Pyralid	Common
65.	*Protostica gravelyil* Laidlaw	Moth	Pyralid	Common
		FAMILY–CHLOROCYPHIDAE		
67.	*Rhinocypha* (*Heliocypha*) *bisignata* (Selys)	Teak pyralid moth	*Hapalia machaeralis* (Walk)	Rare

Contd...

Table 5–Contd...

Sl.No.	*Dragonfly Species*	*Prey*		*Occurrence*
		Common Name	*Scientific Name*	
	ANISOPTERA DRAGONFLIES			
	FAMILY–GOMPHIDAE			
68.	*Gomphus* sp.	–	Unknown	Common
69.	*Gomphus nigricicus* Laidlaw	Mahogany moth	*Hypsiphla robusta* Moore	Common
70.	*Burmagomphus laidlaw* Fraser	Pink borer	*Sesamia inferens*	Common
71.	*Burmagomphus pyramidalis* Laidlaw	Pink borer	*S. inferens*	Common
72.	*Davidioides martini* Fraser	Mosquito	*Anopheles* sp.	Common
73.	*Mesogomphus lineatus* (Selys)	Mosquito	*Culex*	Rare
74.	*Lamelligomphus malbarensis* (Fraser)	Noctuid moth	*Plecoptera* sp.	Rare
75.	*Megalogomphus superbus* Fraser	Jassid	*Empoasca* sp.	Rare
76.	*Cyclogomphus ypsilon* Selys	Mosquito	*Culex* sp.	Rare
77.	*Cyclogomphus heterostylus* Selys	Mosquito	*Cluex* sp.	Rare
78.	*Asiagomphus nilgiricus* (Laidlaw)	Cane moth	*Emmalocera depresella* Swin.	Rare
79.	*Microgomphus* sp.	Pyralid moths	Unknown	Common
80.	*Microgomphus longistigma* (Fraser)	Midge fly	*Contarinia* sp.	Rare
81.	*Heliogomphus* sp.	Jassid	*Emoasca* sp.	Common
82.	*Macrogomphus annulatus* (Selys)	Mango jassid	*Indioscopus* sp.	Common
83.	*Macrogomphus wynaadicus* Fraser	Mango jassid	*Indioscopus* sp.	Common

Contd...

Table 5–Contd...

Sl.No.	*Dragonfly Species*	*Prey*		*Occurrence*
		Common Name	*Scientific Name*	
		FAMILY–CORDULEGASTERIDAE		
84.	*Chlorogomphus xanthoptera* (Fraser)	May fly	Unknown	Common
85.	*Chlorogomphus campioni* (Fraser)	Mayfly	Unknown	Common
86.	*Onychogomphus nilgiriensis nilgiriensis* (Fraser)	Mosquito	*Culex* sp.	Rare
87.	*Megalogomphus superbus* Fraser	Mosquito	*Culex* sp.	Rare
		FAMILY–AESHNIDAE		
88.	*Anax parthenope* (Selys)	Pyralid moth	*H. machaeralis*	Rare
89.	*Anax immaculifrons* Rambur	Pyralid moth	*H. machaeralis*	Common
90.	*Anax guttatus* Burmeister	Pyralid moth	*H. machaeralis*	Rare
91.	*Anaclaeschna jaspidea* (Brum)	Sawfly	Unknown	Rare
92.	*Gynacantha millaridi* (Fraser)	Pyralid moth	*H. machaeralis*	Rare
93.	*Hemianax ephippiger* (Brumeister)	Jassid	*Empoasca* sp.	Rare
94.	*Oligoaeschna martini* (Laidlaw)	Jassid	*Empoasca*	Rare
95.	*Gynacantha dravida* (Lieftinck)	Mosquito	*Culex* sp.	Rare

Contd...

Table 5–Contd...

Sl.No.	*Dragonfly Species*	*Prey*		*Occurrence*
		Common Name	*Scientific Name*	
		FAMILY–LIBELLULIDAE		
96.	*Macromia indica* Fraser	Mosquito	*Anopheles* sp.	Common
97.	*Macromia flavincia* (Selys)	Mosquito	*Aedes* sp.	Rare
98.	*Macromia flavovittata* Fraser	Mosquito	*Culex* sp.	Rare
99.	*Macromia ellisoni* Fraser	Jassid	*S. sogitella*	Rare
100.	*Macromia ida* Fraser	Jassid	*S. sogitella*	Rare
101.	*Macromia irata* Fraser	Jassid	*S. sogitella*	Rare
102.	*Macromia cingulata* Rambur	Jassid	*N. virescens*	Common
103.	*Epophthalmia vittata* Burmeister	Mosquito	*Culex* sp.	Rare
104.	*Epophthalmia frontalis binocellata* (Fraser)	Mosquito	*Culex* sp.	Common
105.	*Macromidia* sp.	Mosquito	*Culex* sp.	Common
106.	*Idionyx optata* Selys	White fly	*Aleurolobus barodensis* M.	Common
107.	*Hemicordulia asiatica* Selys	Moth	Pyraustid moth	Rare
108.	*Idionyx nadganiensis*	Moth	Pyralid moth	Rare
109.	*Idionyx nilgiriensis*	Moth	Pyralid moth	Rare
110.	*Amphithemis mariae* Laidlaw	Moth	Pyralid moth	Rare

Contd...

Table 5–Contd...

Sl.No.	Dragonfly Species	Prey		Occurrence
		Common Name	Scientific Name	
111.	*Hylaeothemis fruhstorferi* (Karsch)	Moth	Noctuid moth	Common
112.	*Lathrecista asiatica asiatica* (Fab.)	Mosquito	*Culex* sp.	Common
113.	*Cratilia lineata* (Brauer)	Jassid	*Empoasca* sp.	Rare
114.	*Orthetrum sabina* (Drury)	Borers	*C. suppressalis*	Common
115.	*Orthetrum glaucum* (Brauer)	Paddy stem borer	*C. infuscatellus*	Rare
116.	*Orthetrum luzonicum* (Brauer)	Paddy stem borer	*C. infuscatellus*	Rare
117.	*Orthetrum pruinosum neglectum* (Rambur)	Army worm	*Mythimna separata*	Rare
118.	*Orthetrum triangulare triangulare* (Selys)	Maize stem borer	*Chilo partellus*	Rare
119.	*Pontamarcha congener* (Rambur)	Paddy stem borer	*C. infuscatellus*	Common
120.	*Palpopleura sexmaculata sexmculata* (Fabr.)	Mosquito	*Culex* sp.	Rare
121.	*Osthetrum ganeshi* (Mehotra)	Moth	Pyralid moth	Rare
123.	*Brachydiplax contaminata* (Fabricius)	May fly	Unknown	Rare
124.	*Brachydiplax sobrina* (Rambur)	May fly	Unknown	Rare
125.	*Urothemis signata signata* (Rambur)	Jassid	*S. furcifera*	Rare
126.	*Diplacodes trivialis* (Rambur)	Moth	*C. incertulus*	Common
127.	*Diplacodes nebulosa* (Fabricius)	Paddy borers (Moth)	*C. incertulus*	Common

Contd...

Table 5–Contd...

Sl.No.	*Dragonfly Species*	*Prey*		*Occurrence*
		Common Name	*Scientific Name*	
128.	*Indothemis limbata sita* Campion	Paddy borers (moth)	*C. suppressalis*	Rare
129.	*Orthetrum taeniolatum* (Schneider)	Paddy borers (moth)	*C. suppressalis*	Rare
130.	*Orthetrum chrysis* (Selys)	Pyralids	*C. suppressalis*	Rare
131.	*Agriocnemis pigmata* (Rambur)	Pyralids	*C. suppressalis*	Rare
132.	*Crocothemis servilia servilia* Drury	Paddy borer	*C. incertulus*	Common
133.	*Neurothemis tullia tullia* (Drury)	Paddy moth	*C. suppressalis*	Common
134.	*Neurothemis intermedia atlanta* Ris	Jassids, Moths	*Empoasca, Chilo* spp.	Rare
135.	*Neurothemis intermedia intermedia*	Paddy jassid	*N. virescens*	Common
136.	*Brachythemis contaminata* (Fabricius)	Paddy moths	*S. inferens*	Common
137.	*Neurothemis flavia* (Drury)	Jassid	*S. furcifera*	Rare
138.	*Diplacodes trivialis* (Rambur)	Paddy jassid	*S. furcifera*	Rare
139.	*Diplacodes nebulosa* (Fabricius)	Jassid	*S. furcifera*	Rare
140.	*Acisoma panorpoides panorpoides* Rambur	Moths	Pyralid moth	Rare
141.	*Trithemis kirbyi kirbyi* Selys	Moths	Pyralid moth	Rare
142.	*Trithemis aurora* (Burmeister)	Paddy Burmeister	Unknown	Common

Contd...

Table 5–Contd...

Sl.No.	*Dragonfly Species*	*Prey*		*Occurrence*
		Common Name	*Scientific Name*	
143.	*Trithemis festiva* (Rambur)	Paddy jassid	*N. virescens*	Common
144.	*Trithemis pellidinervis* Kirby	Paddy jassid	*N. virescens*	Rare
145.	*Onychothemis testacea ceylanica* Ris	Midge	*Contarinia* sp.	Rare
146.	*Rhyothemis variegata variegata* (Linnaeus)	Moths	*H. machaeralis*	Rare
147.	*Hydrobasilieus croceus* (Brauer)	Mosquito	*Culex* sp.	Rare
		FAMILY–CORDULIDAE		
148.	*Tramea basilaris burmeisteri* Kirby	Mosquito	*Culex* sp.	Rare
149.	*Pantala flavescens* (Fab.)	Paddy borers, Paddy leaf eaters	*Chilo* spp., *Nephotettix* spp.	Common
150.	*Hemicordulia asiatica* Selys	Mosquito	*Culex* sp.	Common
		FAMILY–GOMPHIDAE		
151.	*Asiagomphus nilgiricus* (Laidlaw)	Moth	*H. machaeralis*	Common

Sympetrum frequens against the larvae at *Anopheles sinensis* in laboratory and reported that when the nymph size increased, subsequently the number of mosquito larvae consumption also intensified. They also reported the predator prey relationship between *Sympetrum frequens* and the larvae of *Anopheles sinensis* in rice field near Omiya. In Japan Urabe *et al* (1986) revealed that the density of mosquito larvae increased when the nymphal density of the predator becomes low. The distribution patterns of the predators and prey in the smaller field had a non-overlapping tendency, indicating effective predation.

A good example known about dragonflies have been used successfully through augmentative release (AR) is the introduction of half grown larvae of the libellylid *Czocontenemis servilia* into domestic water storage containers in Yangon (Rangoon) in Myanmar (Burma). The water storage containers were used by the aquatic stages of the yellow fever mosquito *Aedes aegypti,* which was responsible for the transmission of dengue fever in that locality. More than 92 per cent of the local population of *A. aegypti* was occupying the containers, which because of their function were easily accessible to householders and control operators. The systemic release of dragonfly larvae during the monsoon season (the time when dengue fever was being transmitted by the mosquito) rapidly depressed the mosquito populations to a level lower than that could have been achieved by any other known method including treatment by chemical insecticide. Sebastian *et al.* (1990) demonstrated the trials of effectiveness of this approach. The Rangoon trial was very much successful, due to fact that both the adults and larvae of dragonflies were effective for controlling the population of mosquitoes as like conventional pesticide. Review of literature clearly indicates that dragonflies are not widely used in pest management programmes inspite of their tremendous potential. Therefore, efforts should be made to utilize more species of dragonflies in management of pest insects.

Bibliography

Ali, S. 1981. The Himalaya in the Indian Ornithology. In the Himalayas: Aspects of Change, p.p. 16-31, edited by J.S. Lall, New Delhi: Oxford University Press, pp. 481.

Ananthakrishnan, T.N. 1978. Impact of deforestration and monoculture plantation on insect fauna of Western Ghats. *Proc. Seminar on Ecodevelopment of Western Ghats;* 1986, 238-243.

Ananthakrishnan, T.N. 1993. Biological diversity concepts and conservation strategies. *Hexapoda;* 5, 5-8.

Andrew R.J., 2002. Egg chorionic ultrastructure of the dragonfly, *Tramea virginia. Odonatologica;* 31(2), 171-175.

Andrew, R.J. and Tembhare D.B. 1993. Structure and development of the internal male reproductive organs in the dragonfly *Tranea virginia* (Rambur). *Funct. Devp. Morphol.;* 3, 121-127.

Andrew R.J. and Tembhare, D.B. 1994. Functional morphology and development of the primary external genitalia of the male dragonfly, *Tranea virginia* (Rambur). *Ann. Entomol.;* 12, 57-62.

Andrew R.J. and Tembhare, D.B. 1996. Surface ultra structure of Egg Chorion of *Bradinopyga germineta* (Rambur) and *Rhyothemis veriegata* (Linn.). *Frascria (N.S.)* 3: 1-5.

Andrew R.J. and Tembhare, D.B. 1997. Collection of Odonata from Nagpur city, Maharashtra State, India. *Fraseria (N.S.)*; 4, 1-4.

Anonymous, 1999. Maharashtra State Gazetteer: Satara District, pp. 35.

Asahima, S. 1949. New dragonflies from Japan, *Insecta Matsum*; 17, 28-34.

Asahima, S. 1951. New dragonflies from North-eastern Asia, Kontyu; 19, 15-22.

Asahima, S. 1961. Description of dragonfly larvae from Darjeeling. Kontyu; 29, pp.240-246.

Asahima, S. 1963. Notes on three dragonfly species. *Akitu*; 11, 21-22.

Asahima, S. 1967. A revision of the Asiatic species of the damselflies of the Genus Ceragrion (Odonata–Agrionidae). *Jap. Journ. Zool.*; 15, 255-334.

Asahima, S. 1973. South Vietnam Odonata taken by Mr. Y. Inoue. *Jap. J. Zool.*; 16, 1-18.

Asahima, S. 1976. A revisional study of the genus *Mnais* (Odonata, Calopterygidae) VIII. A proposed taxonomy of Japanese Mnais Tombo, Tokyo; 19, 2-16.

Asahima, S. 1981. A revision of the Himalayan dragonflies of the genus *Cephalaeschna Bull. Natn. Sci. Mus.*; 7(2), 57-77.

Asahima, S. 1994. Assamese and Burmese *Coeliccia* species in the collection of Dr. Erich Schmidt (Odonata: Platycnemididae) *Trans. Shikoku. Ent. Soc.*; 16: 1-9.

Atkins, M.D. 1980. Introduction to Insect behaviour. PPCI, New York, pp. 1-237.

Ayyar and Ayyar, 1938. On the ecological history of the Western Ghats. *Abstract*, pp. 98.

Baijal, H.N. and J.P. Agarwal 1955. Opsucula Libellulogica I. *Agra Univ. J. Res. Sci.*; 4(2), 453-470.

Beeson, C.F.C. 1941. Ecology and control of forest insects of India and the neighbouring countries Government of India (1961 Reprint), pp. 767.

Bhasin, G.D. 1953. Odonata (In Roonwal, M.L. *et al*, 1953. A systematic catalogue of the main identified collection at the FRI, Dehradun, Parts 9-21) Indian Forest Leaflet; 121(3): 63-69.

Bhoje, P.M. and Sathe T.V. 2003. Faunistic studies on butterflies from Radhanagari Wild Life Sanctuary, India. *Indian J. Environ.* and *Ecoplan.*; 7(3), 655-658.

Bose, G. and T.R. Mitra, 1976. The Odonata Fauna of Rajasthan. *Rec. Zool. Surv. India*; 71, 1-11.

Brauer, F. 1869. Beschreibung neuer Nuropteren aus dem Museum Godeffroy in Hamburg. *Verh. Zool-bot. Wien*; 19, pp. 9-18.

Cannings, S.G., R.A. Cannings and R.J. Cannings 1991. Distribution of the dragonflies (Insecta: Odonata) of the Yukon Territory, Canada, with notes on ecology and behaviour. Royal British Columbia Museum Contributions to Natural Science; 13, 1-26.

Champion, H.G. and Seth, S.K. 1968. A revised survey of the forest type of India. Manager of Publications, Delhi, pp. 404.

Chandrasakhara, C.S. 1984. Western Ghats Development Programme: Approach to the Seventh Five Year Plan 1985-90, pp. 10-19.

Chao, H.F. 1947. On the systematic position, nymphal characters and new species of the genera *Megalestes* and *Sinolestes* (Odonata). *Biol. Bull. Fukien Univ.*; 6, 15-25.

Chao, H.F. 1962. A study of Navasian types of Chinese dragonflies (Odonata). *I. Acta. ent. Sin.*; 11, 24-31.

Corbet, P.S. 1662. A Biology of dragonflies, Witherby, London.

Corbet, P.S. 1980. Biology of Odonata. *A. Rev. Ent.*; 25, 189-217.

Corbet, P.S. 1999. Dragonflies behaviour and ecology of Odonata. Cornell University Press, New York.

Dasgupta, J. 1957. Cytological studies on the Indian dragonflies. *Proc. Zool. Soc. Calcutta*; 10, 1-65.

Davies, D.A.L. and P. Tobin, 1985. The dragonflies of the world: a systematic list of the extant species of Odonata Vol. 2, *Anisoptera. Societas Internationalis Odonatologica Rapid Communications (Supplements)* 5:i-xi, 1-151.

Dreze, J. and Sen, A. 1955. India: Economic development and social opportunity. New Delhi: Oxford University Press, pp. 291-292.

Fabricius, J.C. 1793. Libellula, 2: 373-383 (in Entomologiae Systematicae. Hafniae, Proft. 8).

Fabricius, J.C. 1798. Libellula, pp. 283-286 (in supplementum Entomologiae Systematicae. Hafniae. Proft. and Storch 8).

Fraser, F.C. 1918. Indian dragonflies, Part III. *J. Bombay nat. Hist. Soc.*; 26, 141-171.

Fraser, F.C. 1919a. Indian dragonflies Part IV. *J. Bombay nat. Hist. Soc.*; 26, 488-517.

Fraser, F.C. 1919b. Indian dragonflies, Part V. *J. Bombay nat. Hist. Soc.*; 26, 734-744.

Fraser, F.C. 1919c. Notes on some new and other Indian dragonflies. *J. Bombay nat. Hist. Soc.*; 26, 874-878.

Fraser, F.C. 1920. Indian dragonflies Part 8. *J. Bombay nat. Hist. Soc.*; 27, 253-269.

Fraser, F.C. 1921a. Ibid. Part 9. *J. Bombay nat. Hist. Soc.*; 27, 492-498.

Fraser, F.C. 1921b. Ibid. Part 10. *J. Bombay nat. Hist. Soc.*; 27, 673-691.

Fraser, F. C. 1921c. A list of dragonflies from Mahabaleshwar. *J. Bombay nat. Hist. Soc.*; 27, 540-544.

Fraser, F.C. 1922a. Indian dragonflies. Part 12. *J. Bombay nat. Hist. Soc.*; 28, 481-499.

Fraser, F.C. 1922b. Ibid. Part 13. *J. Bombay nat. Hist. Soc.*; 28, 610-620.

Fraser, F.C. 1922c. Ibid. Part 14. *J. Bombay nat. Hist. Soc.*; 28, 899-910.

Fraser, F.C. 1922d. New and rare Odonata in the pusa collection. *Mem. Deptt. Argic. India* (*Ent.*); 7, 39-77.

Fraser, F.C. 1923. Indian Dragonflies Part 15. *J. Bombay nat. Hist. Soc.*; 29, 36-47.

Fraser, F.C. 1924a. Report on a collection of dragonflies (Odonata) from the Andaman Islands. *Rec. Indian Mus.*; 26, pp. 409-414.

Fraser, F.C. 1924b. A survey of the Odonata (Dragonfly) Fauna of Western India with special remarks on the genera *Macromia* and *Idionyx* and description of thirty new species. *Rec. Indian Mus.*; 26, pp. 423-522.

Fraser, F.C. 1925a. Indian dragonflies. Part 20. *J. Bombay nat. Hist. Soc.*; 30, 397-405.

Fraser, F.C. 1925b. The true position of the genera *Orogmphus* and *Chlorogomphus* as demonstrated by a study of the larvae of *O.*

atkinsoni and *O. cmpioni* and by a comparison of the latter with the larva of *Anotogaster nipalensis* (Odonata). *Rec. Indian Mus.*; pp. 423-429.

Fraser, F.C. 1925c. Indian dragonflies. Part XXI. *J. Bombay nat. Hist. Soc.*, 30: 657-663.

Fraser, F.C. 1925d. Indian dragonflies. Part XXII. *J. Bombay nat. Hist. Soc.*, 30: 846-857.

Fraser, F.C. 1926a. Indian dragonflies. Part XXIII. *J. Bombay nat. Hist. Soc.*, 31: 158-171.

Fraser, F.C. 1926b. Indian dragonflies. Part XXIV. *J. Bombay nat. Hist. Soc.*, 31: 408-426.

Fraser, F.C. 1926c. Dragonflies A Revision of genus *Zygonyx* Selys. *J. Bombay nat. Hist. Soc.*, 31: 763-769.

Fraser, F.C. 1927.a Indian dragonflies. Part 27. *J. Bombay nat. Hist. Soc.*; 32, 183-196.

Fraser, F.C. 1927b. Ibid. Part 28. *J. Bombay nat. Hist. Soc.*; 32, 311-319.

Fraser, F.C. 1928. Indian dragonflies. Part 29. *J. Bombay nat. Hist. Soc.*; 32, 450-459.

Fraser, F.C. 1929a. Ibid. Part 32. *J. Bombay nat. Hist. Soc.*; 33, 288-301.

Fraser, F.C. 1929b. Ibid. Part 33. *J. Bombay nat. Hist. Soc.*; 33, 576-597.

Fraser, F.C. 1929c. Ibid. Part 34. *J. Bombay nat. Hist. Soc.*; 33, 834-850.

Fraser, F.C. 1930. A new Indian dragonfly (Order: Odonata) *J. Bombay nat. Hist. Soc.*; 34, 752-735.

Fraser, F.C. 1931. Additions to the survey of the Odonata (Dragonfly). Fauna of Western India with descriptions of nine new species. *Rec. Indian Mus.*; 33, 443-474.

Fraser, F.C. 1932. Indian dragonflies. Part XXXIX. *J. Bombay nat. Hist. Soc.*; 35, 645-656.

Fraser, F.C. 1933. The Fauna of British India. Odonata. Taylor and Francis, London, I, xiii+420 1 map.

Fraser, F.C. 1933, 1934 and 1936. The Fauna of British India including Ceylon and Burma. Odonata, 1: xiii+ 423 pp., 2: xxiii + 398 pp., 3: xi+461 pp. Taylor and Francis, London.

Fraser, F.C. 1934. The Fauna of British India, Odonata, Taylor and Francis, London; II, xxiii+398, 10 pls.

Fraser, F.C. 1935. New Oriental dragonflies (Order: Odonata). *Rec. Indian Mus.*; 37, 321-333.

Fraser, F.C. 1936. Fauna of British India including Ceylon and Burma. *Odonata*, 3, Taylor and Francies Ltd., 461 pp.

Fraser, F.C. 1940. A comparative study of the genes of the family Gomphidae (Order: Odonata). *Trans. R. ent. Soc. London*; 90, 541-550.

Gadekar, R.R., Chandrasekhara, K. and Nair, P. 1990. Insect species diversity in the tropics, sampling methods and a case study. *J. Bombay nat. Hist. Soc.*; 87, 353-357.

Gadgil Madhav 1981. Dams, Hills and Forests, in major dams a second look, pp. 12-20.

Gadgil Madhav and Meher Homjo, V.M. 1986. Role of protected areas in conservation; in conservation for protective agriculture. Ed. Chopra VIL and T.N. Khoshoo (New Delhi, Indian Council of Agricultural Research) pp. 143-159.

Gaonkar, H. 1996. The butterflies of Western Ghats, India and Srilanka. A biodiversity assessment on the ecological history of Western Ghats. Abst., pp. 90.

Ghosh, A.K.; Biswas, S.; Lahiri A.R. and Rynth M.R. 1975. Some records of insect fauna of Manas Wild Life Sanctuary. *Sci. and Cult.*; 41, pp. 386-388.

Goldsmith, E. and Hildyard, N. 1984. The Social and Environmental effects of large dams volume one-overview. Wadebridge Ecological Centre, Worthyvale, U.K.; pp. 346.

Imms, I.D. (1963). A general text book of Entomology, APH, New Delhi.

IUCN 1980. World Conservation Strategy: Living resource conservation for sustainable development. IUCN, Gland, Switzerland.

Jalan, B. 1996. India's Economic Policy: Preparing for the 21st Century, New Delhi: Penguin Books, pp. 217.

Joseph, K.J. 1984. Insect life and ecodevelopment of the Western Ghats. *Proc. Seminar on Ecodevelopment of Western Ghats*, 1986, pp. 84-89.

Joseph, T.M. 2004. Biodiversity conservation in the Western Ghats: Biodiversity and Environment, 17, 221-227.

Joseph, J. and I. Satyarani, 1988. On a small collection of Odonata from Andhra Pradesh, India. *Rec. Zool. Surv. India;* 85, pp. 439-450.

Khoshoo, T.N. 1995a. Census of India's Biodiversity takes ahead. *Curr. Sci.,* 69: 14-17.

Khoshoo, T.N. 1995b. Census Biodiversity takes ahead. *Curr. Sci.,* 69: 14-17.

Kiauta, B. 1975. Cytotaxonomy of dragonflies with special reference to the Nepalese Fauna, X+ 76 Nepal Research Centre, Kathmandu.

Kimmins D.E. 1966. A list of Odonata types described by F.C. Fraser now in British Museum (Natural History). *Bull. Brit. Mus. (Nat. His.) Ent.;* 18, 173-227.

Kimmins D.E. 1968. A list of the type specimens of Libellulidae and Cordullidae (Odonata) in the British Museum (Natural History). *Bull. Brit. Mus. (Nat. His.) Ent.;* 22, 277-305.

Kimmins, D.E. 1969. A list of the type specimens of Odonata in British Museum (Natural History). Part II. *Bull. Brit. Mus. (nat. His.) Ent.;* 23, 287-314.

Kulkarni, P.P.; D.B. Bastawade and S.S. Talmale 1999. Predation of dragonflies *Ictinogomphus rapax* (Rambur) and *Pantala flavescens* (FABK) (Odonata: Anisoptera), By the Giant wood spider, *Nephila maculata* (FABR.) Vol. 1(4).

Kulkarni, P.P. and Prasad M. 2002. Insecta: Odonata Zool. Surv. India: Wetland Ecosystem Series No. 3: Fauna of Ujani, 91-104.

Kulkarni, P.P.; M. Prasad and Talmale, S.S. 2002. New record of damselfly *Pseudagrion microcephalum* (Rambur) from Maharashtra (Odonata: Coenagrionidae). *Bionotes;* 4(3), 58.

Kumar, Anil 1990. Odonata of Vedanthangal waterbird sanctuary, Tamil Nadu, with notes on their field ecology. *J. Bombay nat. Hist. Soc.;* 87, 320-323.

Kumar, A. and T.C. Khatri 1985. On a small collection of Dragonflies (Odonata) from the Eastern Ghats, Tamil Nadu, Uplands-1. *Eastern Ghat Insecta;* 1, 6-9.

Lahiri, A.R. 1975. Note of the behaviour of *Bayadera hyalina* Selys in the rain (Zygoptera: Euphaeidae), *Odonatologica*, 4, pp. 255-257.

Lahiri, A.R. 1976. Colicnemia mukherjeei, sp.n. from Khasi hills India (Zygoptera: Platychemididae). *Odonatologica*; 5, pp. 273-276.

Lahiri, A.R. and S. Das 1991. Observation on the epicranio-orbital complex of some Indian Aeshinae (Odonata: Aeshnidae). *Rec. Zool. Surv. India*; 89(1-4), 155-166.

Laidlaw, F.F. 1902. On a collection of dragonflies made by members of the Skeat expedition in the Malay Peninsula in 1899-1900. *Proc. Zool. Soc. London*; 1, 63-92.

Laidlaw, F.F. 1914. Odonata. Zoological Results of the Abor Expedition 1911-1912. *Rec. Indian Mus.*; 8, 335-349.

Laidlaw, F.F. 1915a. Notes on Oriental dragonflies in the Indian Museum No.1. *Rec. Indian Mus.*; 11, 197-199.

Laidlaw, F.F. 1915b. Odonata Fauna of Chilka lake. *Mem. Indian Mus.*; 5, 178-180.

Laidlaw, F.F. 1916a. Notes on oriental dragonflies in the Indian Museum No.4. The genus Pseudagrion *Rec. Indian Mus.*; 12, 21-25.

Laidlaw, F.F. 1916b. Notes on Indian Odonata subfamily Agrionidae, Genus Ischnura Charp, Genus Ceriagrion Selys; subfamily Gomphinae, Genus Davidius Selys. *Rec. Indian Mus.*; 17, 129-139.

Laidlaw, F.F. 1917a. A list of the dragonflies recorded from the Indian empire with special reference to the collection of the Indian Museum. Part I. Family Calopterygidae. *Rec. Indian Mus.*; 13, 23-40.

Laidlaw, F.F. 1917b. A list of the dragonflies recorded from the Indian empire with special reference to the collection of the Indian Museum. Part II. Family Agrionidae. *Rec. Indian Mus.*; 13, 321-348.

Laidlaw, F.F. 1919. A list of the dragonflies recorded from the Indian empire with special reference to the collection of the Indian Museum. Part II. Family Agrionidae (contd.) *Rec. Indian Mus.*; 16, 169-195.

Laidlaw, F.F. 1920. A list of the dragonflies recorded from the Indian Empire with special reference to the collection of the Indian Museum Part III. *Rec. Indian Mus.*; 19, 145-163.

Laidlaw, F.F. 1921. A list of the dragonflies recorded from the Indian Empire with special reference to the collection of the Indian Museum. *Rec. Indian Mus.*; 22, 75-91.

Laidlaw, F.F. 1922a. A list of the dragonflies recorded from the Indian Empire with special reference to the collection of the Indian Museum. The subfamily Gomphinae. *Rec. Indian Mus.*; 24, 367-426.

Laidlaw, F.F. 1922b. A list of dragonflies recorded from the Indian empire with special reference to the collection of the Indian Museum Part IV. The subfamily Gomphinae. *Rec. Indian Mus.*; 24, 361-414.

Laidlaw, F.F. 1924. Notes on oriental dragonflies of the genus Aciagrion.. *Proc. U.S. Nat. Mus.*; 66(Art 10), 1-9.

Laidlaw, F.F. 1930. A synonymic list of dragonflies of the family Gomphidae (Order: Anisoplera) found in the oriental region. *Trans. R. ent. Soc. London*; 78, 171-191.

Laidlaw, F.F. 1932. A revision of the genus Coeliccia (Order: Odonata). *Rec. Indian Mus.*; 34, 7-42.

Lieftinck, M.A. 1948. Odonata. Entomological Results from the Swedish Expedition 1934 to Burma and British India. *Arkiv. For Zoologi.*; 41A No, pp. 1-23.

Lieftinck, M.A. 1953. Additions to the Odonate fauna of the Indo-Australian Archipdago. *Treubia*; 22, 233-269.

Lieftinck, M.A. 1960. On the identity of some little known Southeast Asiatic Odonata in European Museums described by L. de Selys Longchamps with descriptions of new species. *Mem. Soc. ent. Ital.*; 38, 229-256.

Lieftinck, M.A. 1968. A review of the Genus *Oligoaeschna* Selys in South east Asia. *Tijdschrift voor Entomologic deel 111 afl.*; 5, pp.137-184.

Lieftinck, M.A. 1969. Two new Odonata from South East Asia comments on previously described species. *Dt. ent. Z*; 16; 205-21.

Lieftinck, M.A. 1977. New and little known Corduliidae (Odonata: Amisoptera) from the Indo-Pacific region. *Oriental Ins.*; 11, pp. 157-179.

Mani, M.S. 1993. Modern Classification of Insects Pub. Satish Book Enterprise, Moti Matra, Agra, India pp.1-331.

Martin, R. 1908-1909. Aeschnines, pp. 1-223. (in collections zoologiques du Baron Edm. de Selys Longchamps 18-20, Institut royal des Sciences naturelles du Belgique, Brussels).

Martin, R. 1909. Aeschnines. *Cat. Coll. Selys Fasc.*; 19, 85-156.

Mathew, G. 1982. A survey of beetles damaging commercially important stored timber in Kerala KFR Research Report 10, Kerala Forest Research Institute, Peechi, pp. 92.

May, E. 1933. Odonatologische Mitteilungen. VI-VIII. *Senckenbergiana*; 17, 97-218.

Mclachlan R. 1895. Some new species of Odonata of the Legion Lesters with notes *Ann. Mag. nat. Hist.*(6), 16, 19-28.

McLachlan, R. 1896. On odonata from the province of Szechuen, in Western China and from Moupin in Eastern Tibet. *Ann. Mag. Nat. Hist.*; 17(6), 364-374.

McNeely, J.A.; Miller, K.R.; Reid, W.V.; Mittermeier R.A.; Werner T.B. 1990. Conserving the Worlds' Biodiversity, Washington, DC: World Resource Institute, pp. 193.

Mitra, T.R. 1983. A list of Odonata of Calcutta. *Ent. mon. Mag.*; 119, 29-31.

Mitra, T.R. and G.C. Sen 1975. First records dragonflies (Odonata: Anisoptera) from Tripura (India). *Ent. Rec. J. Var.*; 87, 119-120.

Mohan Kumar B. 2006. Woodfuel resources in India. *Proc. Nat. Acad. Sci. India*, 76(B) (1), 1-9.

Moore, N.W. 1997. Dragonflies: Status Survey And Conservation Action Plan. IUCN/SSC Odonata Specialist Group. pp. 27.

Mukhopadhay Koushik, Ranjan bera, Ratneswar ray 2005. Modern Agriculture and Environmental Pollution. *Evergman's Science*; 11(3), 186-192.

Nair, N.C. 1984. Conservation of botanical resources of the Western Ghats from a taxonomical points of view. Paper presented in workshop on Ecodevelopment of Western Ghats, Trivendrum, 11-13 May, 1984.

Nair, K.S.S.; Mathew G. and Sivarajan M. 1981. Occurrence of the bagworm *Pterowea plagiophleps* Hampson (Lepidoptera: Psychidae) as pest of the tree *Albizia falcataria* in Kerala, India. *Entomon.*; 6, 179-180.

Navas, R.P.L., 1930-1934. Insectos de la India. *Rev. Acad. Cienc. Zaragoza*; 13, 29-31 (1930); 15 11-41 (1932); 29-33 (ano 1933, 1934).

Needham, J.G. 1930. A manual of the Dragonflies of China. *Zool. Sinica Ser. A.*; 11, 346+11.

Needham, J.G. 1932. A key to the dragonflies of India, *Rec. Indian Mus.*; 34, 195-228.

Pachauri, R.K. and Shridharan, P.V. 1998. Green India 2047, looking back to think ahead. *Green India*; 31, 1-346.

Pandharbale, A.R. and Sathe, T.V. 2001. On a new species of the genus *Syntomis* (Syntomidae: Lepidoptera) from the environment of Western Ghats (Satara District. *Indian J. Environ.* and *Ecoplan.*; 5(3), 601-602.

Pandharbale, A.R. and Sathe, T.V. 2002. Abundance and distribution of the moths: families Noctuidae, Sphingidae and Syntomidae from Western Ghats and plain region of the Satara district (Maharashtra). International Conference of SAARC countries on Biotechnology in Agriculture, Industry and Environment, 2002, Karad, India, Abstr.

Pinhey, E.C.G. 1974. A revision of African *Agriocnemis* Selys and *Mortonagrion* Fraser (Odonata: Coenagrionidae). *Occ. Pap. nat. Mus. Rhod*, 85, 171-178.

Prasad, M. 1974 Odonata of Garhwal Hills. *Bull. Ent.*, 15, 41-55.

Prasad, M. 1976a. Odonata of district Kangra (Himachal Pradesh). *Rec. Zool. Surv. India*, 71, 95-119.

Prasad. M. 1977b. Report on the collection of dragonflies from Punjab, India, Part. I. *Newsl. Zool. Surv. India*, 3, 309-312.

Prasad, M. 1995. On a collection of Odonata from Goa, India. *Frasseria*, (N.S.); 2(12), 7-8.

Prasad, M. 1996. An account of the Odonata of Maharahstra State, India. *Rec. Zool. Surv. India*; 95(3-14), 305-327.

Prasad, M. 1999. Faunal diversity in India: Odonata. *Zool. Surv. India, Calcutta*; pp. 171-178.

Prasad, M, and Kumar, A. 1977a. Extension of distribution of some dragonflies (Odonata) in Western Himalaya (U.P.) *Newsl. Zool. Surv. India*, 3, 170-174.

Prasad, M. and Varshney, R.K. 1995. A check-list of Odonata of India including data on larval studies. *Oriental Ins.*; 29, 385-428.

Prasad, M. and P.P. Kulkarni 2001. Insecta: Odonata Zool. Surv. India: Fauna of Conservation Area Series 11: Fauna of Nilgiri Biosphre Reserve: pp. 73-83.

Prasad, M. and P.P. Kulkarni 2002. Insecta: Odonata. Zool. Surv. India: Fauna of Eravikulam National Park. *Conservation Area Series* No.; 13, 7-9.

Prasad, M. and R. K. Thakur 1981. Further additions to the Odonata (Insecta) from Rajasthan. *Janyu*; 1, 26-28.

Prasad, M. and R.K. Vershney 1988. The Odonata of Bihar, India. *Rec. Zool. Surv. India Occ. Pap. No.*; 110, 1-47.

Prasad, M. and S.K. Ghosh 1984a. A note on the Odonata (Insecta) from Khasi Hills, Meghalaya with description of a new species. *Bull. Zool. Surv. India*; 6, 37-44.

Prasad, M. and S.K. Ghosh 1984b. A note on the Odonata (Insecta) from Sikkim, India, *J. Bombay nat. Hist. Soc.*; 80, 435-438.

Prasad, M. and Singh, A. 1976. Odonata of Doon Valley. 2. Zygoptera *Rec. Zool. Surv. India*, 70, 121-131.

Prasad, M.; P.P. Kulkarni and S.S. Talmale, 2000. New record of andromorphic females in two species of Neurothemis dragonflies (Odonata: Libellulidae) from Central India. *Bionotes*; 2(3), pp. 54.

Prasad, M.; Ram, R. and Ghosh, S.K. 1987. Notes on the Indian species of the Genus *Pseudagrion* Selys (Coenagrionidae: Odonata). *Bull. Zool. Surv. India*, 8(3): 313-321.

Prasad Rajendra 2005. Towards sustainable agriculture in India. *Natl. Acad. Sci. Lett.*; 29 (1&2), 41-44.

Pyle, *et al*, 1981. Insect Conservation. *Ann. Rev. Ent.*; 26, 233-258.

Ram, R.; V.D. Srivastava and M. Prasad 1983. A note on a collection of Odonata from eastern Uttar Pradesh, India. *Notul. Odonatol.*; 2, 15-16.

Rambur, M.P. 1842. Histoire Naturella des Insectes. Nevropteres. xvii-534 pp. Librairie Encyclopedique de Roret, Paris.

Rao, K.R. and A.R. Lahiri 1982. First records of Odonata (Arthropoda: Insecta) from Silent Valley and New Amarbalom reserved forests. *J. Bombay nat. Hist. Soc.*; 79, 557-562.

Ravindranath, N.H. and Hall, D.O. 1994. Indian forest conservation and Tropical deforestation (synopsis). *Ambio.*; 23(8), 521-523.

Ris, F. 1909. Libellulinen. 2. *Cat. Coll. Selys Fasc.*; 10, 120-224.

Ris, F. 1910. Libellulinen. 3. *Cat. Coll. Selys Fasc.*; 11, 244-384.

Ris, F. 1911. Libellen Von Sintang, Borneo gesammelt von Dr. L. Martin. *Ann. Soc. Ent. Belg.*; 55, 231-255.

Ris, F. 1912. Neue Libellen von Formosa, Sud China, Tonkin and den Phillippenen. *Mitl. Suppl. Ent.*; 1, 44-85.

Ris, F. 1912. Uber Odonaten Van Java Und Krakatau. *Tijidschr. Ent.*; 55, 157-183.

Ris, F. 1913. Odonata von den Aru and Kei Inseln gesammelt durch Dr. H. Merton 1908 nebst Ubersicht under die von den Aru-Inselnbekannten Odonaten. *Abh. Senckenb. Aru. Lenda naturforsch. Ges.*; 34, 501-536.

Ris, F. 1916. Sewter's Formosa–Ausbeute *Odonata Suppl. Ent.*; 5, 1-81.

Rodger, W.A. and Panwar, H.S. 1988. Planning of wildlife protected area network in India-1 and 2 Dehra Dun. Wildlife Institute of India.

Roonwal, M.L. 1953. On a new evolutionary phenomenon: The sharp increase of intraspecific variation in minimum populations as evidenced by the Desert Locust. *Symp. Organic evolution* (March 1953) *Abst. (Nat. Ins. Sci. India)*; pp. 10-11.

Sahni, D.N. 1964. Survey of the Insect Fauna of Nainital (Odonata) Anisoptera. *Agra Uni. J. Res.* (Sci.); 13, 89-98.

Sahni, D.N. 1965. Studies on the Odonata of Nainital Indian. *J. Ent.;* 27, 205-216, 277-287.

Sahni, D.N. 1972. Studies on the Odonata of Kumaon. Part I. Suborder Anisoptera, family Libellulidae. *Bull. Ent. Soc. India;* 11, 37-54, 121-130.

Sathe,T.V.2004. *Vermiculture and Organic Farming.* DPH, New Delhi pp. 1-216.

Sathe, T.V. 2005. Impact of dragonflies on population suppression of paddy pests in agroecosystem of Kolhapur, India. *Proc. 4th WDA Int. nat. sym. Odonatology* spain (July 2005).

Sathe, T.V. 2006. Biological Control of Mosquitoes *Proc. Mat. Sym. Rec. Trend Malarial Studies,* Pune pp. 11-17.

Sathe, T.V. and P.M. Bhoje, 2000. *Biological Pest Control,* DPH, New Delhi. pp. 1-122.

Sathe, T.V. and Y.A. Bhosale, 2001. *Insect Pest Predators.* DPH, New Delhi pp. 1-169.

Sathe, T.V. and G. S. Margaj, 2001. *Cotton Pests and Biocontrol Agents.* DPH, New Delhi pp. 1-166.

Sathe, T.V. and Pandharbale A.R. 1999. Hawk moth (Sphingidae: Lepidoptera) diversity in Western Maharashtra including Ghats. *Geobios;* 18, 77-82.

Sathe, T.V. and A.R. Pandharbale 2005. Biodiversity of Moths (Order: Lepidoptera) from Western Ghats of Satara district, India. *Bull. Biol. Sci.* 1, 81-88.

Sathe, T.V. and K.P. Shinde 2006. Diversity of butterflies from Western Ghats (Kolhapr district). *J. Natcon.* 18(1), 181-184.

Sathe, T.V. and Shinde K.P. 2006a. On a new species of the genus *Rhyothemis* Hagen (Order: Odonata) from India. *J. Nat. Con.,* 18(2), 421-424.

Sathe, T.V. and K.P. Shinde 2006b. On a new species of the genus *Agriocnemis* Selys (Order: Odonata) from India. *J. Curr. Sci.,* 9(2), 799-802.

Sathe, T.V., K.P. Shinde, B.V. Jadhav and T.M. Chougale 2006. Role of dragonflies for suppression of pests in mulberry ecosystem in Kolhapur, India. *Proc. Asia. Pacif. Cong. Seri* and *Insect Biotech.,* Korea (S) (52), 159.

Sathe, T.V. 2005. *Basic Entomology: A Practical Manual.* DPH, New Delhi, pp. 1-118.

Sathe, T.V. 2006. Biological Control of Mosquitoes *Proc. Mat. Sym. Rec. Trend Malarial Studies*, Pune. pp.11-17.

Sathe, T.V., Inamdar, S.A. and Santakumar, M.V. 1986-87. Fauna of Butterflies from Western Maharashtra and Western Ghats (Part of Maharashtra only), India. *J. Shivaji Uni.* (Science); 23, 391-398.

Sathe, T.V. and Pandharbale, A.R. 1999. Hawk moth (Sphingidae: Lepidoptera) diversity in Western Maharashtra including Ghats. *Geobios;* 18, 77-82.

Sathe, T.V. and Pandharbale, A.R. 2001. On a new species of genus *Syntomoides* Hampson (Lepidoptera: Syntomidae). 71st Annual Session, The National Academy Sciences, Pune, India, October, 5 to 7, 2001 Abstr. 20, pp. 30.

Sathe, T.V. and Pandharbale, A.R. 2004. Biodiversity of moths from Western Ghats of Satara district, Maharashtra. *Int. Nat. Workshop on Recent Trends in Environmental Sciences*, New Delhi. Abts.

Sathe, T.V. and A.R. Pandharbale 2005. Biodiversity of Moths (Order: Lepidoptera) from Western Ghats of Satara district, India. *Bull. Biol. Sci.;* 1, 81-88.

Sathe T.V. and K. P. Shinde 2006. Diversity of butterflies from Western Ghats (Kolhapur District). *J. Natcon.*, 18 (1), 181-184.

Sathe, T.V., Shinde Kiran; Bhoje, P.M.; Thite, H.S., 2005. Biodiversity of dragonflies (Odonata) from Western Ghats of Maharashtra, India. 4th *WDA International Symposium of Odonatology.* Poentevedra, Spain, 26-30th July, 2005 (presented).

Sathe, T.V., Bhoje, P.M.; Kavane, R.; Shinde Kiran, Yadva, R.P. and Pandharbale, A.R. 2005. Mating behaviour in a damselfly *Ischnura sengalensis* (Rambur). 4th *WDA International Symposium of Odonatology.* Poentevedra, Spain, 26-30th July, 2005 (presented).

Satish, P.M. 1996. Moths and Butterflies of Bhadra Project. M.Sc. Thesis submitted to Kuvempu Univeristy, Shimoga, pp. 80.

Schmidt, E. 1938. Check-list of Odonata of Oceania. *Ann. ent. Soc. Amer.;* 31, 322-344.

Schmidt, E. 1951. The Odonata of Madagoscar. Zygoptera. *Mem. Inst. Sci., Madagascar*; 6A, 115-283.

Selys, Longchamps, E. De 1859. Additions au Synopsis des calopterygines. *Bull. Acad. Belg. Sci.* 7, 437-443.

Selys, Longchamps, E. De. 1889. Odonates de Sumatra. *Ann. Mus Civ. Stor. nat. Giacomo Doria, Gemova*, 7, 444-484.

Selys, Longchamps, E. De. 1891. Odonates de Birmanie. *Ann. Mus. Civ. Stor. nat. Giacomo Doria Genova*; 10, 433-518.

Sharma, R.M.; S.S. Talmale and P.P. Kulkarni 2000. Odonates attracted to light at Tadoba-Andhari tiger Reserve, Maharashtra, 2(1).

Shinde, Kiran 1989. Impact of dam construction and agricultural practices on the animal diversity in the Koyna catchment. M.Phil. thesis. Shivaji University, Kolhapur.

Shinde, K.P. and Sathe, T.V. 2006. Biodiversity of dragonflies (Odonata) from Koyna dam and around area. *16th All India Congress of Zoology and national Symposium on recent advances in animal research with special emphasis on invertebrates. Proc.* 52.

Singh, S. 1955. Entomological survey of the Himalayas Part V. On two new species of Odonata. *Agra Univ. J. Res. Sci.*; 4, 171-174.

Singh, S. and H.N. Baijal 1954. Entomological survey of the Himalayas II. On a collection of Odonata. *Agra Univ. J. Res. (Sci.)*; 3, 385-400.

Singh, S.; H.N. Baijal; V.K. Gupta and K. Mathew 1955. Entomological Survey of the Himalayas. Part XIV Notes on some insects collected by the Second entomological expedition to the North West Himalays (1955) with description of three new species of Odonata. *Agra Univ. J. Res. (Sci)*; 4(suppl), 741-744.

Singh, A. and M. Prasad, 1974. New records of Odonata from North-West India. *J. Bombay nat. Hist. Soc.*; 70, 403-405.

St. Quentin, D. 1937. Neue Odonaten aus Assam. *Konowia*; 16, 85-89.

Sushil Kumar 2005. Prospects for sustainable agricultural production of the antimalarial molecule artemisinin in India. *Science letters*; 28 (9 and 10), 325-338.

Talmale, S.S. and P.P. Kulkarni, 2003. Odonata in paddy fields of Bhandara district, Maharashtra. *Bionotes*; 5(3), 67.

Tembhare, D.B. 1979. Hormonal regulation of osmotic and ionic balance in the haemolymph of the larvae of dragonfly *Aeschna cyanea* (Muller). *Arch. Internat. Physiol. Biochim.*; 87, 557-563.

Tembhare, D.B. and Thakare, V.K. 1977. Neurosecretory system of the ventral ganglia in the dragonfly, *Orthetrum chrysis* (Selys). *Cell. Tiss. Res.*; 177, 269-280.

Thakare, V.K.; Tembhare, D.B.; Khan, M.W. and Pendharkar, V. 1980. Chemical composition of haemolymph in the larvae of the dragonfly *Orthetrum chrysis* (Selys). *Odonatologica*; 9, 32-324.

Tillyard, R.J. 1916. Life histories and descriptions of Australian Aeschninae, with a description of a new species of Teleophlebia by Herbert Campion. *J. Linn. Soc. Zool.*; 33, 1-84.

Tillyard, R.J. and Fraser, F.C. 1938-1940. A reclassification of the order Odonata. *Aust. Zool.*; 9, 125-169; 195-221; 359-396.

Tyagi, B.K. 1984. List of odonata of the Chandigarh Union territory on the Chandigarh Siwalik out crops. *India, Notul. Odonatol.*; 2, 61-62.

Vershney, R.K. 1971. On some dragonflies of Khasi hills. *J. Assam. Sci. Soc.*; 14, 97-100.

Williamson, E.B. 1904. The dragonflies (Odonata) of Burma and Lower Siam. I. Subfamily, Calopteryginae. *Proc. U.S. nat. Mus.*; 28, 165-187.

Williamson, E.B. 1907. The dragonflies (Odonata) of Burma and lower Siam-II. subfamily Cordulegasterinae Chlorogamphinae, Gomphinae, *Proc. U.S. nat. Mus.*; 33, 317.

Wright, S. 1932. The roles of mutation in breeding, cross breeding, and selection in evolution. Proc. 6th Int. Cong. Genet (Ithaca); 1, 356-366.

Wyber-Blyth, M.A. 1957. Butterflies of Indian Region. *Bom. Nat. Hist. Soc.*, Bombay, 1-523.

ZSI–Zoological Survey of India, 1983. Threatened Animals of India, Zoological Survey of India, Calcutta, pp. 307.

Index

www.ingramcontent.com/pod-product-compliance
Ingram Content Group UK Ltd.
Pitfield, Milton Keynes, MK11 3LW, UK
UKHW020207290926
15470UKWH00001B/46

9 789351 240037